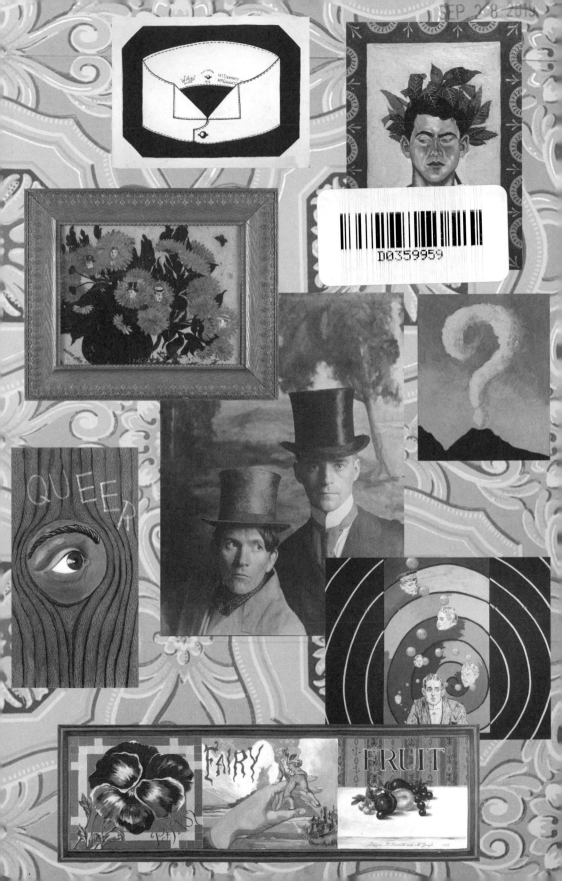

QUEER

FAIRY FRUIT

I've Seen the Future and I'm Not Going

I've Seen the Future and I'm Not Going

The Art Scene and Downtown New York in the 1980s

PETER McGOUGH

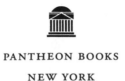

PANTHEON BOOKS

NEW YORK

Library of Congress Cataloging-in-Publication Data
Name: McGough, Peter, [date] author.
Title: I've seen the future and I'm not going: the art scene and downtown New York in the 1980s / Peter McGough.
Description: First edition. New York: Pantheon, 2019.
Identifiers: LCCN 2018060306 (print). LCCN 2019000228 (ebook).
ISBN 9781524747053 (ebook). ISBN 9781524747046 (hardcover).
Subjects: LCSH: McGough, Peter, [date]. Artists—New York (State)—
New York—Biography. AIDS (Disease)—Patients—New York (State)—
New York—Biography. Gays—New York (State)—New York—Biography.
Classification: LCC N6537.M39656 (ebook).
LCC N6537.M39656 A2 2019 (print). DDC 700.92—dc23
LC record available at lccn.loc.gov/2018060306

www.pantheonbooks.com

Front-of-jacket photograph by Josef Astor
Jacket design by Janet Hansen
Endpapers: all paintings are by McDermott & McGough;
all photographs are by Peter McGough.

Printed in the United States of America
First Edition
2 4 6 8 9 7 5 3 1

For Stella Schnabel and Mike Meagher

Wisdom rises on the ruins of folly.

—THOMAS FULLER

Acknowledgments

I would like to thank my editor, Shelley Wanger, for her endless patience and tireless help in shaping this book. I am forever grateful to Luke Janklow for suggesting I write my memoir in the first place and to my agent, Emma Parry, for encouraging me at the beginning and subsequently every step of the way.

I could never have done a proposal without the guidance and vision of Eve Claxton and Lizzie Jacobs or the generous support of Alison Gingeras and Piotr Utlanski. I am emormously grateful to Senior Production Editor Kevin Bourke and to Patrick Dillion for his meticulous research and copyediting.

To my friends and family, thank you for your support and encouragement: Mark Arena, Jason Arbuckle, Josef Astor, Allisa Bennet, Jeannette Montgomery Barron, Aileen Corkery, Scott Covert, Wouter Deruytter, Hugo Guinness, Miciah Hussey, Jean Kallina, Michael Kors, David Macke, Elizabeth MacKenzie, Mary Bergtold-Mulcahy, Ryan Ouimet, Jack Pierson, Philip Ramus, John Richardson, Jacqueline Schnabel, Margaret Seiter, and Kate Simon. And last, but not least, many thanks to Ivaylo Gueorgiev for his heroic work on the art and photo research for the book.

I wrote this memoir as I remembered this time in my life. I never kept a journal and there may be parts others will remember differently, but these are stories my friends and I have shared for years.

I've Seen the Future and I'm Not Going

Prologue

The worst part of being sick, truly sick, was the night. I'd shoot awake from a searing pain that started in my toe and ran right up the inside of my leg. Within seconds my whole limb was on fire. After about twenty minutes, the pain would subside, but now I was wide awake. I'd lived in Manhattan for most of my adult life, but until I was up nightly, I had never realized how quiet Times Square could be at three in the morning: a stillness that left me defenseless against the crushing thoughts of the past and its glory, and of my present dire circumstances.

It was 1998, I was on the good side of forty, and I was almost dead. Paul Bellman, my doctor, the man who was known for pulling patients off the edge of doom, later told me that when he saw me for the first time, he thought, "This person has three months to live." I didn't know it, but his treatment plan wasn't to cure me, which looked impossible even to a man considered one of the best AIDS doctors in the world; his plan was simply to make me comfortable in my final weeks.

A few friends and ex-assistants came to visit. I could tell by their startled faces I must have looked a wreck. I was a skeletal one hundred pounds, covered from head to toe in purple, AIDS-related Kaposi's sarcoma sores, with my once thick mane of blond hair now wispy and thin. I greeted my guests in a frayed nightshirt as I sank into a foot-high feather mattress in my antique brass bed, made for McDermott and me by Iskobel Iskowitz, where I spent my days and sleepless nights. The bed was one of the few remnants from my days of grandeur.

Even if I wanted to leave my apartment—which I rarely did—I could barely manage the stairs. Without savings or livelihood, I was living in the only place I could afford: a glorified attic, five crooked flights of stairs above Forty-Sixth Street in Midtown Manhattan—"Little Brazil"—in a slanting nineteenth-century town house. And, for the first time in my adult life, I was living alone.

Only a few blocks away from the stone lions of the stately New York Public Library, the street floor of this once grand house was now a Japanese restaurant for the lunchtime business crowd. From my sickbed at night I could hear the rats fighting over the scraps of mid-priced sushi in the back garden. The second floor had a Brazilian hair salon that specialized in bikini waxing. The sexy Latino proprietor would stand in the window with his uniform of skintight black jeans and a form-fitting dark T-shirt, overseeing the needs of his clients and his coterie of beautiful assistants. The third floor was an "Asian Beauties" massage parlor. I painted a sign and taped it to my door that read, WHORES ON 3RD FLOOR! DON'T BOTHER TO KNOCK!, to stop the familiar, soft tapping from their late-night clientele. After a raid closed the massage parlor I broke the police lock and chain on the door to see what was there. The Victorian ornament around the ceiling, now crumbling, was painted black like the walls and the indoor/outdoor–upholstered cube where clients waited for attention. I peeked into the sad little single rooms where men would get massaged. As though frozen in time after the raid, there were still large plastic bottles of economy-sized body lotion and rumpled sheets. At the end of the hallway was a washer/dryer that had stopped in midwash amongst a pile of dirty sex towels. A bok choy dish was still on a dirty hot plate, and melted votive candles were strewn about the soggy-carpeted floor.

Above this pleasure palace, on the fourth floor lived a thin, pale artist, Chivas Clem, who had told my friend Jane Rosenblum about the apartment. I could always tell when it was eleven a.m. because his alarm clock would ring for an hour while he was in deep, medicated slumber. Chivas was the director of the Pat Hearn art gallery, aka PHAG, in Chelsea. It was one of the first three galleries to move from SoHo to Chelsea, along with Matthew Marks and Morris-Healy. I showed with Pat in the eighties when she was in the East Village. After Pat's death in 2000 her husband, Colin de Land, took over the gallery space.

Chivas's apartment also doubled as a gallery he called "the Fifth International," where he put on exhibitions. One evening Chivas heard me in the hallway and invited me in for a drink. I noticed the remains of drugs on an overturned *Artforum* magazine with an ad for my former Swiss art dealer, Bruno Bischofberger. Chivas was just finishing dinner with two young artists on the rise, Rob Pruitt and Elizabeth Peyton. I stayed a bit to be polite and begged forgiveness for leaving so soon. I couldn't bear how embarrassed I felt about how far I had fallen and that my looks foretold how ill I was.

In my fifth-floor apartment above Chivas I had a kitchen and three large rooms which I painted in blue, green, and white to hide the cracks and cheap plaster repairs. I didn't have any furniture but my bed, so I borrowed two rooms of antique furniture from my friend Ricky Clifton who was decorating artists' apartments. I promised to buy them but kept putting him off because I could barely make the rent. I set up a white-walled painting studio in the front parlor with the easel and art supplies my friend Walter Fleming bought me and where—when I had the strength to get out of bed and my bedroom—I started to paint again. The rest of the time I painted from my bed, finishing watercolors for a show in Paris.

My bedroom was in the back, where I could see a jeweler (the Diamond District was the next block) working diligently through the night, his room illuminated by the blue flames of his trade. My friend Mary Bertold from FIT was so horrified after seeing where I lived and how I looked that she bought me a small refrigerator, which she had her friend

Liz drag up the five flights so I could keep food there. Mary would burst into tears with each visit or phone call. A lot of people cried when they visited. I felt terrible that I upset them.

"How the hell did I end up here?" I'd sigh at night as the fumes of burning flesh filled the apartment from the fast-food burger place below. I had watched so many friends die miserable deaths from AIDS and now my number was up. I felt damned and cursed. As I passed people on the streets I wanted to change lives with any of them. I'd take their lot. Anything was better than this death sentence.

Only a little more than a decade before, in 1986 a painting I made with my partner, David McDermott, was on the cover of *Artforum*, at the time the international bible of the art world; and in 1993, a picture of us and our assistants in our studio was the cover of *Art in America*. We had sold-out shows in the best galleries in New York and Europe and endless invitations to museum openings, art parties, society events, and movie premieres. Our life was seemingly a never-ending one of fame and luxury.

After the financial crash in 1987 we lost our 1840s town house on Avenue C in the East Village, lit by candlelight and heated by fires in the hearths. We had filled the two floors above an old storefront with mid-nineteenth-century antique furnishings right down to the drinking glasses. Our mattresses were foot-high striped ticking, fluffed into mountains full of feathers. We covered the cracked walls in period papers and hung vintage prints, paintings, and mirrors for our nineteenth-century "time experiment." Every object had to fit perfectly—no modern element was allowed there, not even a telephone. As a part of our time machine, we wore detachable starched collars and cuffs, high-button shoes, silk top hats and capes, and carried walking sticks—among our vast period wardrobe.

We also lost our studio in 1994 which had been the Kings County Savings Bank, an intact 1865 three-story Second Empire limestone building on the corner of Broadway and Bedford Avenue in Williamsburg, Brooklyn. We had acquired it in 1989, decades before the arrival of frat boys and Wall Street financiers. The bank's first floor housed our offices that we furnished with period manual typewriters, candlestick telephones, and oak office furniture, all under a grand ceiling lit by six hanging cast-iron early electroliers. At noon each day a chef would arrive with a vegetarian lunch to feed the staff. Our British secretary, Jane, also wore period antique clothes. We forbade our studio assistants to wear printed T-shirts and had them wear smocks while they worked, to cover their modern dress. The second floor was our sun-filled painting studio, with many assistants stretching and preparing the canvases. And above that was our photography studio, with a twenty-three-foot-high ceiling and pumpkin-colored walls piled high with our antique props, period costumes, and large wooden view cameras. There we published the one issue of our magazine, *The Cottage, Protector of Hearth and Home,* and had it printed in New York with a hand-set letterpress.

But perhaps what I missed the most was our "miniature mansion," as we called it: an untouched brick house from 1790 with no heating, plumbing, or electricity. The only heat source was the fireplaces, where we cooked our meals, and the water was from a hand-pump well outside the kitchen door. The house was next to an 1880s general store with an apartment above it and a Greek Revival two-seater outhouse with wallpapered walls. It was set among tree-shaded barns and a carriage house alongside a flowing stream in Oak Hill, in the Catskills.

We also gave up our 1913 crank Model T Ford touring car, our 1926 Model A truck, and a plush navy-colored 1930 Graham-Paige luxury car with silk window shades, a bud vase, and a brass blanket bar for the backseat. Not to mention our horses, carriages, handmade saddles and riding boots. After the IRS seized our property, they had a three-day auction in Albany of all the antique furnishings of the house, the general store, the apartment above it and the contents of the barns. I begged the local antiques dealers, whom I knew well, and those who came from far and wide, not to bid against us, so I could buy back the contents of my life. My pleas fell on deaf ears. The highest bidders left with our furnishings, eighteenth-century clothes, carriages, and an 1880s wooden, horse-drawn omnibus with a Hudson River scene painted on the side which held eighteen passengers. All that remained were our feather mattresses and a few old American flags since they couldn't sell them legally. I had to remind them of that fact.

McDermott departed for Ireland in the summer of 1994, on the *QE2* with a one-way ticket his grandmother bought him, saying he wanted to live in a country that protected its artists. At that point Irish artists didn't have to pay taxes. I thought he'd return after a year, but he didn't—and that was how years later I found myself living alone in a fifth-floor walkup off Times Square, trying to stay alive and revive our floundering career.

"If only I had kept McDermott under control," I uttered to no one.

1

I was always a shy child, with a fear of strangers and unfamiliar places, and from an early age I was a target of school bullies. My mother, Susan, encouraged my interest in art by enrolling me in drawing and watercolor classes in Syracuse, where we lived in a suburb. She was friendly and kind—her Catholic faith was a big part of her life—but she also had a scary temper. Suddenly she'd come running out of a room with a large wooden spoon or my father's army belt for a harsh lashing. I'd be livid after the beating and not speak to her for as long as possible. I once watched a 1950s B horror movie called *The Wasp Woman,* about a cosmetics queen who is transformed into a murderous monster—part female, part wasp—who pounced on her victims as they screamed in horror and then dragged them out of the room. That movie terrified me as a child. That's how I saw my mother, a good-looking, sweet woman who had uncontrollable rages and too many children. I was one of seven, the fifth oldest with three sisters and three brothers.

My parents were generally good people and the nuns at school would say, "Your mother's a saint." But when her fury of a temper appeared, I tried to run as fast as I could and hide upstairs till the storm had passed. If it wasn't directed at me, it was at one of my sisters or brothers. Then one day the army belt went missing. I can't even begin to understand how difficult it was to have a child every year with no help and little if any rest, plus a husband who most days was on the road for business.

When I was growing up in the sixties there wasn't much to see in the way of art in Syracuse except the new Everson Museum designed by I. M. Pei. In the seventies Yoko Ono had a show there and she came with John Lennon. And there was a show of Warhol's and Jamie Wyeth's portraits of each other. Making art became my refuge. I lived in a fantasy world of my own making, and with drawing, I could create a place where I felt safe and in control. I'd sketch places of serenity, beauty, and joy: a clown in a hoop, or a beautiful woman walking a clipped poodle down a city street. These sheets of paper were my little

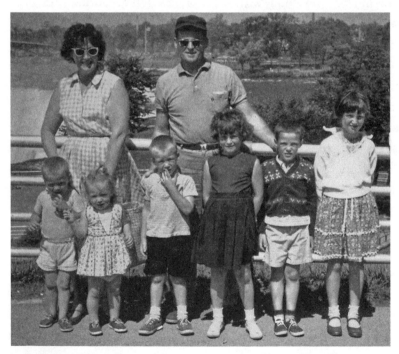

A family trip to Niagara Falls, early 1960s: my mother and father; front row, left to right, me, Margaret, John, Beth, Tommy, and Mary Susan

kingdom of people and places where I wouldn't be interrupted with a slap or an insult.

Our all-white suburban neighborhood had four different-style houses that the owners could choose from and have built. They came with a small tree on the front lawn and a backyard. As I grew older and was allowed to freely roam the streets of infinite sameness, I noticed that the blocks of houses went from the 1950s style, like the one we lived in, all the way back to the forties, thirties, twenties, then the teens and oughts.

I had first heard the term "colored person" as a child. In my naive ignorance I thought it was someone covered in different hues of green, yellow, and purple. When I actually saw a black person in the flesh it was in my mother's front parlor. She was giving a tea with the local parish priests, using her best china and silverware, for a black priest visiting from Nigeria. I was introduced, smiled, and then was sent out of the parlor to go play in the yard. Debbie, the girl next door, came up to me, saying, "Your mother's a nigger lover." The next thing I knew, my younger sister Margaret was jumping on Debbie, yanking Debbie's scarf tightly around her neck. I pulled her off as Debbie ran crying to her house. After the honored guest from Nigeria and the other priests left, Debbie's mother came to our back door and reprimanded my mother about our behavior. My mother turned to us and made us apologize. We were horrified by this demand but obeyed after she refused to let us tell our side of the story. When she left, my mother said we were to pray for them. Years earlier, the father had blown his brains out with a shotgun in his bedroom, and the mother's son ended up in prison in the seventies for selling drugs, with the serial killer the Son of Sam as his cellmate.

My parents were active Catholics in their local cinderblock church in the shape of a crucifix up the hill from the cinderblock shopping mall. My mother was one of a group of ladies who cleaned the altar or baked bread for the homeless. My father, Tom, was a Sunday-school teacher who also brought bibles to prisoners and preached the gospel. I never heard any derogatory remarks from them against any other race or religion. Everyone was equal in God's eyes, I was told. Except for one group, the homosexuals. "You know how your father feels about homosexuals," my mother would inform me.

When I first asked her what a homosexual was, she told me, "They're sad and lonely people who don't know if they're a man or woman." And this was from someone who had never met one. I could sense her fear that I was one with such remarks as "If you go out dressed like that, then they'll really call you a fruit." With my limited wardrobe of my two older brothers' hand-me-downs, I somehow still looked fruity? I must have, since sometimes my father would address me by the name Shirley, probably to keep me from acting too swish. It didn't work. I was just being myself, but these words stung. Was I a bad person because of my attraction to the other boys? I didn't think there was anything wrong with me, and I didn't pray to be changed. But I knew I had to keep this a secret. I also suspected something was up with my mother by her reactions to what I would try to watch on TV. One afternoon, I was settling in to the movie *Days of Wine and Roses,* with Lee Remick and Jack Lemmon as alcoholics, when she came into the room and ordered me to turn it off, and after I protested she went up to the TV and did it herself. Another time a news program was doing a segment on child molestation. She demanded that I switch channels. The same went for *The Naked Civil Servant,* a film with John Hurt playing the flamboyant homosexual Quentin Crisp. It wasn't just about her being protective, but rather her own issues. She had this odd answer when she didn't want to talk about a subject: "Ask me no questions and I'll tell you no lies."

It was my sister who clarified matters when she told me our mother had recently figured out from birth records that she was a "love child" and that her parents were forced to marry. Our mother's father was an Irishman who had the "drinking curse." Her parents were servants from Scotland who worked in the big houses in Main Line Philadelphia. Bessie, my grandmother, was a cook; my grandfather was the butler. Gran's sister, Helen, was the nanny and her red-headed husband, Ben, was another butler. I remember Ben was walking me to the beach in Avalon, New Jersey, one summer, and as we stopped by a cottage with a sign that said WEE BUTTON BIN (meaning the size of a button box) over the door, my granduncle touched my shoulder to get me to look up at him. I must have been nine, and he said, "Don't ever become a servant, son. It's a horrible, horrible life—working for pennies for the wealthy." When I was older, my mother would tell me a story about how her parents lost their jobs due to my grandfather's drinking. His employers would find him passed out drunk in their parlor. In the Great Depression my mother and her sisters, Tessie and Lizzy, were sent over to Scotland to live with Granny Cairns; her own parents were to follow—until the relatives there said the poverty was worse in Scotland and to stay in America. My mother slept with her adored Granny Cairns and her other two sisters in a bed in the kitchen. Her uncle and cousins were across the room in a bed sleeping four abreast. The rest of the family slept upstairs. Years later, when I was living in Dublin and she came to visit, I suggested we go to Scotland to visit where she came from. "No," she replied, "I have enough memories." I felt for her having such parents, an alcoholic father and the harsh taskmistress Bessie. To see my mother cower in front of her mother, wanting her approval, was saddening.

Bessie was bossy and highly critical. When she was coming to visit, my mother would get hysterical trying to clean up the house. "Susan—your house is out of order! . . . Susan—your children are running wild! . . . Susan—get ahold of yourself! . . . Susan—you've gained weight again." Gran was tough and expected everyone to live up to her standards. On the other hand, my father's mother, Mamie, a tiny redhead gone white, was lovely. "Look at your beautiful drawing," she'd say to me, or "What a lovely singing voice you have!" Mamie had moved to America during the Easter Rising in Ireland and left her tiny eighteenth-century home with its rose garden. When I was in Dublin, at the foot of the Royal Hospital, which is now a museum, I would look over the stone wall of her abandoned house and see the roses she often spoke of still in bloom among the brambles and weeds.

Decades later, at Bessie's wake (she died at 102), my mother burst into tears at the casket. That sobbing turned into a howl of pain. My heart ached at the sight. Her deep sobbing connected all the dots of their relationship for me. Like my mother, I have my secrets, my fears, and my rage but keep a façade of what she would call "nicey-nice," a role perfected to hide pain and loss. I'm very much my mother's son.

I have a vivid memory of my father on the phone in the kitchen begging the bank not to take our house as my mother stood frozen, wringing her hands. My father lost his job in Syracuse because when asked to get "girls" for the visiting executives from out of town, he refused. My father told them, "I don't pimp for anyone." That day he came home, I was sick and in front of the television. As usual he took off his hat and put it on the closet shelf, hung up his overcoat, and placed his briefcase on the floor below the coats. My mother sat in silence in the kitchen, holding a cup of tea. When I asked why he was home so early that day, he replied, "I lost my job." He then went into their bedroom with my mother and closed the door.

My mother was very encouraging about my art, and even with our meager financial resources she always found money for art supplies. I feel she was the one who made me into an artist. When I was a teenager and wanted to become an actor, she discouraged me and advised me to continue with art. I always felt she was saying to me, "You don't belong in a place like Syracuse, you have to get out." My sister Beth became an art teacher, but the rest of them took normal jobs. I was never interested in sports or other things boys are supposed to be interested in. "I don't want realism. I want magic," as I heard Blanche DuBois say. I was always looking for a protector who would rescue me from the straight life. Where was that life I saw on TV?

By high school my wardrobe became my statement. I bought a favorite belted wrap sweater at the shop Tops and Bottoms down the hill at the cinderblock mall because it reminded me of the one Mari-

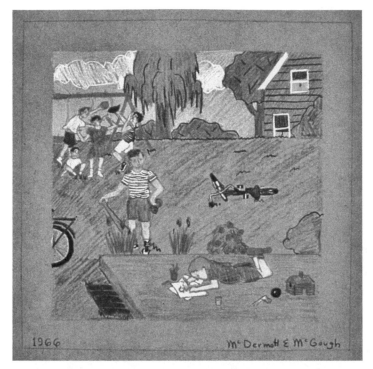

A crayon drawing by David and me on butcher-block paper for our last show at Massimo Audiello's gallery. I am drawing on our patio, ignoring the pleas to play sports.

lyn Monroe wore in a beach photo. I was obsessed with her. I would always check the paper's weekly TV schedule to see if any of her films were playing. With only one old television in a house of nine family members, I had to carefully plan any takeover of the television. What I found so alluring about Monroe, aside from the way she looked and spoke, was her brilliant sense of comedy, but even as a kid I felt there was something else. She had that lost, vulnerable look in her eyes. She seemed so insecure, just like I felt. I remember riding the school bus one day after I had just seen Kim Novak in *Vertigo* on TV the night before. I thought about her character's vulnerability and how she had two personalities. Judy was the real person, a cheap brunette who lived in a single-room-occupancy hotel, and Madeleine, the rich, sophisticated blonde. I felt like her characters in that I also had something to hide. I wanted to be with those women I saw in old films on TV. When they cried, I cried. As they waited by the phone for their blasé lover to call, I waited with them. Though I adored these women I didn't want a girlfriend. Nor did I want to be a woman. I wanted my English teacher, and I joined the gymnastics team just to be near him, his black hair and mustache. Once I stupidly gave him a homemade valentine card. That ended my being on the team.

I have hated waking up early for as long as I can remember. Each weekday morning my father called out our names, from the oldest to the youngest. I dreaded the idea of having to face another day of school. I'd drag myself down for breakfast as my mother was making our lunches. I'd rush to get dressed in my uniform and to catch the school bus that luckily stopped in front of our house. In class I couldn't seem to concentrate. I'd be drawing women's faces in my notebook instead of the lesson on the chalkboard. I also had bullies to avoid.

Ron, my best friend in grammar school, at least I thought so, was a wide door of a person, with a massive head topped off with frizzy white-blond hair that he tried to comb down with a side part. One day in fourth grade I sat down at my usual perfectly organized desk. When I opened it, I found a total mess. Someone had destroyed my carefully arranged papers. I knew it was Ron. I could tell, but I never said anything. On the first day of fifth grade I stood with the cool kids hoping to be a part of their group. I thought I had finally made it from their friendly smiles and questions about my summer vacation. Then Ron accused me in front of the other boys of hanging out with girls the whole summer since he saw me at the mall with my sister and her group of girlfriends. He said he saw me at the makeup counter trying on lipsticks. I was just looking at the lipsticks. Right there and then I knew it was over. I was branded with a capital F for Fag. And my dreams of being friends with the coolest and best-looking boys vanished. Rumors spread fast, and I was left with the other outcasts and big-boned girls.

So, I made the best of it as I slid along the hall lockers trying to avoid punches from the cool boys who were now my enemies.

Unfortunately, I soon realized I had another opponent in the guise of a strongly built redheaded girl named Amber-Anne. Amber-Anne liked to fight, and she always asked me to battle her on the playground at recess. I kept thinking, "She'll tear my clothes—or worse spill my blood—or maybe both!" One day Ron came to school with a terrible sunburn. ("White blonds can't take the sun," my mother told me when I repeated the tale of horror to her.) His sunburn covered his neck and went down his back, glowing through his white poly-cotton shirt. While a nun with a whistle herded us off the playground in two straight lines, boys in one, girls in the other, to return to afternoon class, I watched Amber-Anne raise her hand while she walked in line across from Ron saying, "Hey, Ron, how are ya doing, man?" and letting her palm fall loudly on his back. He let out a pitiful, piercing screech and fell to the concrete sobbing. Some of us in line drew back in horror, while the others laughed at this cruel attack. The nun came over to see what the commotion was. No one dared rat out Amber-Anne, not even her latest victim, who still lay there weeping.

I felt sorry for Ron but I was also somewhat happy watching my burnt-flesh persecutor, and former best friend, writhing in pain on the playground destroyed by my own soon-to-be-annihilator, Amber-Anne. For the next thing I knew, just as we were getting into our assigned seats, she passed by and placed a folded piece of notebook paper on my desk, sneering as she headed back to her desk.

With much trepidation I opened the folded document. I read the crude printing. "WILL YOU FIGHT ME TOMORROW? YES OR NO. CIRCLE ONE." Panic ensued. I hated that I had to answer her demand and return her fiendish missive. I looked over at my redheaded persecutor. She was squinting, staring straight into my ten-year-old heart, nodding as her hand was clenched in rage toward me. She tilted her head and raised one eyebrow that demanded my reply. I knew I had to answer her or else be shamed by the whole class. I looked at my punisher's coterie of female miscreants whispering and giggling as they stared back and forth between us, so as not to miss a scene in this schoolyard drama. One tiny mean girl caught my fear-stricken eyes and let her wrist go limp mocking my feyness. How I wished Amber-Anne would pummel her right there and then, and understand that I was the truly desired friend!

"How can I fight this amazon?" my mind raced. "This devil's twice my size!" But I had to answer her note somehow. I slowly picked up my pen out of the groove in the plastic desktop. I looked at her masculine hand on the scrawled note. "Yes" meant I'd have to lose to her for a life-time of shame all the while surrounded by the others in their blue plaid Catholic uniforms taunting me as I had witnessed others before on the parking-lot playground. "No" meant I was a coward. Surely I *was* a coward! But the other option was that I would be beaten up and still be shamed. I couldn't win either way. "Oh, I hope she doesn't hit me in the face!" I thought. She'd also wreak havoc on my uniform. Then the answer "No" kept resounding in my head. "No, no, no!" But "Yes" was blood and bruises. I looked at her note more intently: YES OR NO. CIRCLE ONE. Shaken, I exhaled deeply and whispered a prayer. Then, out of nowhere, a flash of genius befell me: I circled "Or." I proudly folded the missive and held it out to one of her waiting handmaidens. I watched, trying to read Amber-Anne's face as she went over the note. "She'd have to think it was funny," I said to myself. But before I knew it I was under her massive shadow as she towered above me. I quickly thought of ducking and hiding under my desk. But before I could move I felt the whopping thunder of her fist pound into my arm. My mouth opened with a whimper as I fell in a clump onto the cool linoleum floor, clutching my limb as my eyes smarted with the pain.

At school I had enemies to avoid; on my neighborhood street I had some admirers. My hair had grown to my shoulders into a thick blond mane which the nuns did not approve of. But I was the envy of the neighboring housewives. I would often go down the street and sit with one of them on beach chairs in her driveway. Soon more housewives holding cups of tea or coffee and offering cookies would join us. Days later I read in the "Dear Abby" column about a mother asking for advice about how to tell if her son was a homosexual. Abby answered that one sign would be her son hanging out with a group of women. From then on, I avoided the ladies' coffee klatsch. One day when I was on my bike one of the neighboring ladies stopped me and asked why I wasn't coming by anymore. I made up some excuse, but I was sad because I had really enjoyed our talks.

That summer we called on my rarely visited uncle Bill in Philadelphia. Looking over at my sisters and me, he said to my father, "Tom, I thought you had three daughters, not four." I don't remember my father's reply, but I do remember the look he gave me. Later he took me to a barber and ordered him to cut off all my hair. I didn't put up a fight because I knew the answer could be a lashing. "Now you look like a boy is supposed to," he said later, as we drove home. I didn't reply, I just pressed my head against the car window, looking out as we drove along the highway. Tom, my father, was a good-looking black-Irish jock from Philadelphia who had been the captain of his college and army basketball teams. My eldest brother Tommy, named after my father, was closeted about his sexuality and his drinking. I caught him taking sips from a liquor bottle kept in a lower cabinet in our kitchen when he was about thirteen. I was shocked that he was doing it and he threatened me not to tell on him. He was a kind and quiet person who usually had his face in a book, but he was an alcoholic from an early age, and I remember being frightened when he was in high school and got into a physical fight with my father over his drinking as he stumbled into the house. Eventually, he became sober.

At the end of the summer just before the start of seventh grade, I suddenly didn't feel well. I couldn't run around, and I kept complaining I was sick. "You just don't want to go back to school," my second oldest sister Beth said. Of course, I didn't want to return to the bullying and the boredom. She was right, I hated school with its daily taunting and physical harassment. But I had never felt so ill. I was sitting on the living-room sofa wrapped in a blanket because I was so cold. My mother had called the doctor and he said there was a flu going around and not to worry. When she hung up the phone and came back to see me still slumped on the sofa with my sister Margaret next to me, I screamed, "I have to throw up, I have to throw up!" My mother picked up an old stone pot and dumped out the dry flower arrangement. Then a wave of acid-green vomit spewed out into the pot, on me, and splattered my mother's dress as my sister jumped aside. My mother screamed for my father to get in the car while she quickly bundled me up and put me in the backseat with her as we sped to the doctor's office. After a brief examination, he said to get me to the hospital immediately because my appendix had burst. I must have passed out because the next thing I knew I was being rushed on a gurney through busy hallways to the operating room clutching my mother's left hand and staring at her diamond engagement ring sparkling under the fluorescent lights. Later, I woke up in a hospital room to the tall, handsome priest from our parish reciting Latin prayers as he anointed me with oil. I was being given last rites. With blurred vision, I saw a dark shadow of my parents and could hear my mother softly crying as she prayed along. This was my first experience of being seriously sick and isolated. It would not be my last.

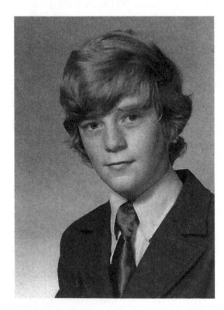

Just out of the hospital: the eighth-grade picture that caused the nickname "Peter Permanent"

For the first few weeks of my six-month stay, I was kept drugged and was in and out of consciousness. There was a second visit from the priest and more Latin prayers and oil. I was put on beds of ice to bring down my temperature and I ended up with pneumonia. A nurse would come in every day and give me many shots in the thigh until it hurt too much. Then the daily shots went in my behind. I looked like a skeleton and all my hair fell out. Then I slowly started to get better. The bandages were changed daily on the hole that had been cut in my right side, which oozed green pus. My nurse was a buxom dark beauty from Eastern Europe who fawned over me. Somehow a baseball game was on my TV set and a curvaceous girl in a bikini ran out onto the field and kissed the pitcher. The nurse was shocked at such a display of flesh and cursed her for being so vulgar. I loved it and thought the bikini beauty was fantastic. My mother came every day while my brothers and sisters were at school. I was in a room with another patient but the TV was on my side (a curtain divided the room) so I could look at old movies and my favorite shows. I had never had such luxury. To my amazement, presents, cards, and flowers kept arriving. Puzzles and game boards and more and more and more—and they were all for *me*! I had never seen such loot. "Now this is living," I thought. I was sharing a room with another child. He died and a new one came in. There was a blind kid who'd push another in a wheelchair down the hall. A beautiful blond jock from my brother's class was across the hallway. He broke his leg playing football. I prayed he would visit me since I was bedridden. Sadly, he didn't.

The nun from my seventh-grade class brought in a white cloth dog with the signatures of all my classmates. I feigned that I didn't feel well so I wouldn't have to speak to her. She had the reputation of being the meanest teacher at school, but she was also quite beautiful from what I could see. "What's she being a nun for when she's so gorgeous?" I thought. The week before, my sister Margaret came and told me the scandal that had the whole school talking. A pretty mean girl in this nun's class came in wearing lip gloss and mascara. The nun ordered her to wash it off with a sponge that was used to clean the blackboards while she stood in front of the whole class. She apparently cried as she washed with the water from the bucket that held the large, dirty sponge. After my initial shock at the nun's heinous sadism, I laughed. That pretty girl always snubbed me. After my mother gave the nun my health report, the nun filled us in on how the class was going on without me: "They miss you," she said, and walked out of the room with my mother as she called out, "The whole class is praying for you!"

"Yeah, right," I thought. I faked a smile and looked over the names on the little dog. Mary, my good and mostly only friend in school, was the first name I spotted. It went downhill from there. And then, there it was, the mark of Lucifer: "AMBER-ANNE," written in ballooned large capital letters. The nerve of that beast! I seethed at her bold name standing among the childish scribbling and threw the dog across the floor. My mother returned and picked it up and looked at me curiously. "It fell," was all that I could say, and I turned on the TV, using the greatest invention ever made in the eyes of this seventh-grader: the remote control.

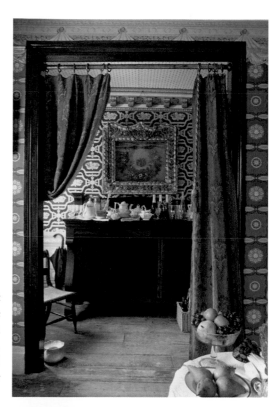

The pantry off the front parlor of our town house at 113 Avenue C, between Seventh and Eighth Streets, which McDermott and I decorated together

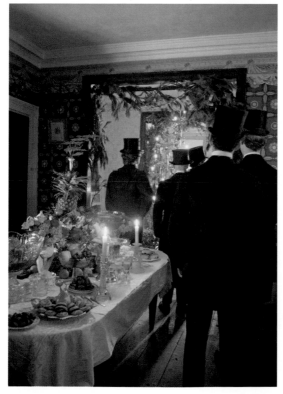

Justin Hoag staged a festive Christmas for a photo shoot at Avenue C; *left to right:* David McDermott, Simon Boden, Justin Hoag, Sebastian, and me.

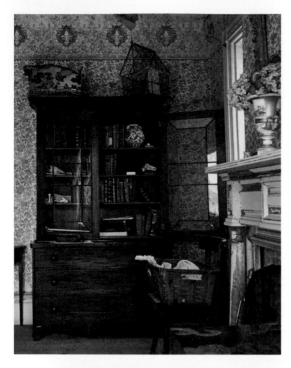

The parlor at Oakhill,
the 1790s brick house that
we bought in 1989, with
its original 1900s wallpaper;
the bookcase was once in the
Thomas Cole house in Catskill.

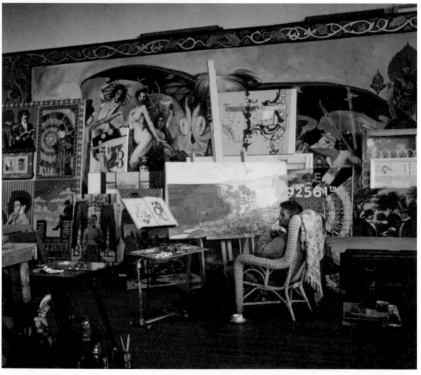

I am sitting on the top floor of the King's County Bank in Williamsburg, which
we had originally used only as our photography studio. In 1994 we started using it
for storage and as a painting studio.

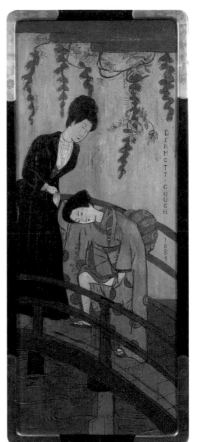

Two Women on a Bridge, 1884, 1983
Oil on linen, 20" x 10"

A Meiji painting from our first
show, in 1983, which was at Ricky
Clifton's North Star Gallery on
Sixth Avenue below Prince Street

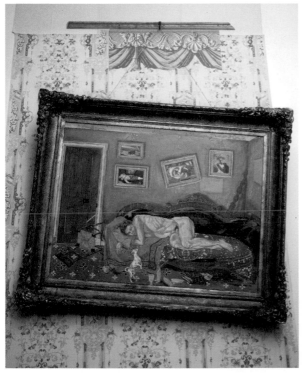

The Scapegoat, 1863, 1985
Oil on linen, 40" x 50" x 4"

From Massimo Audiello's
group exhibition, *The Chi-
Chi Show,* 1985, at his East
Village gallery on Eleventh
Street and Avenue A

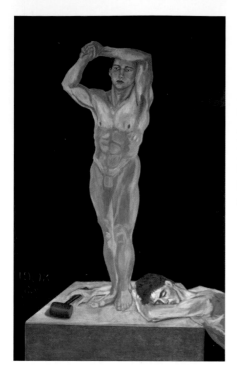

Pygmalion, 1908, 1985
Oil on linen, 48" x 60"

Brian Fleming, our friend
John Patrick's brother, posed for
the statue; Andy Warhol bought
it at the opening of our first
solo show at Massimo's gallery.

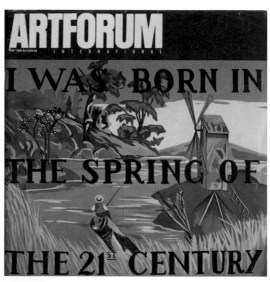

"I Was Born . . ."
Oil on canvas

Our 1986 *Artforum* cover

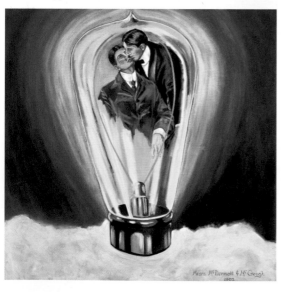

No Arguments, 1903, 1986
Oil on linen, 60" x 60"

The subject was a statement
about our constant arguments.

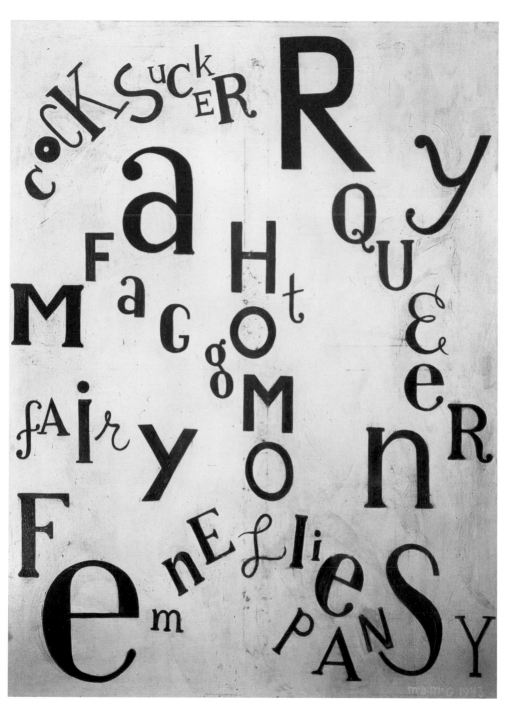

A Friend of Dorothy's, 1947, 1987 Oil on canvas, 76" x 66"

This painting was included in the 1987 Whitney Biennial.

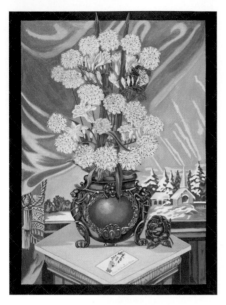

The Flower Painting, 1888, 1987
Oil on cotton, 70 ½" x 50 ½"

Massimo told us to make more
commercial art so I painted the
flowers into a dollar sign.

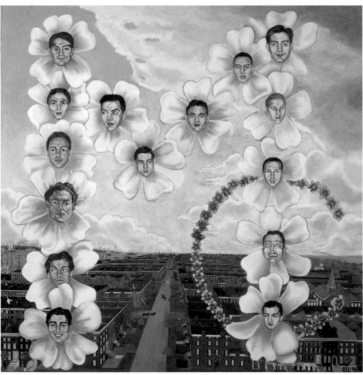

The Daisy Chain, 1889, 1987 Oil on linen, 60" x 60"

A group of our friends with McDermott, top left, and me, top right;
Julian Schnabel is three up on the left. Set against McDermott's idea of
the Lower East Side of Manhattan in the nineteenth century, the daisies
form an "M," and the pansies form a "C" from our last names. Half the
people in this painting died of AIDS.

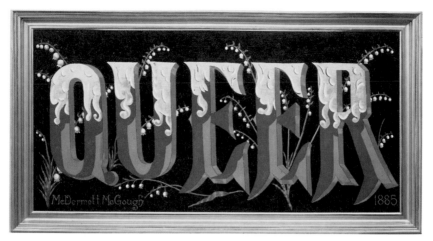

Queer, 1885, 1987 Oil and gold leaf on linen, 44" x 88"

I took a Victorian postcard with a name on it and changed it; I felt I was taking the word from shame to empowerment.

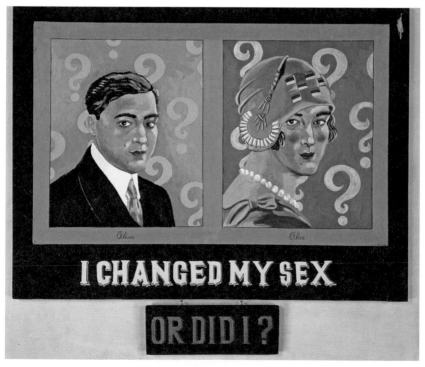

I Changed My Sex or Did I, 1927, 1988 Oil on linen and wood, framed, 27" x 35" x 4"

This was a question that fascinated me.

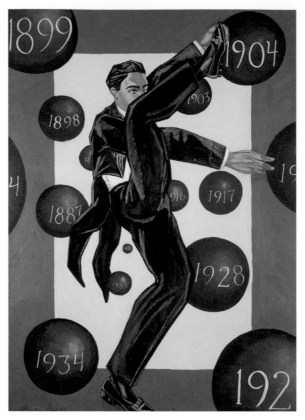

Time Balls, 1921, 1988 Oil on cotton, 51" x 43 ½"

David McDermott dancing through time

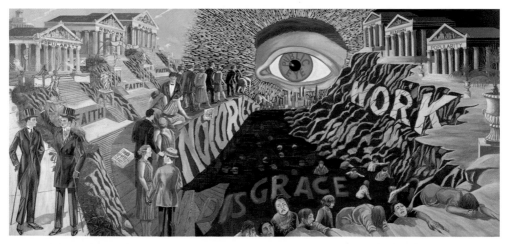

Trying to Get There, 1987 Oil on linen, 72" x 144"

A painting inspired by a 1920s illustration about fame that I saw in Kenneth Anger's book *Hollywood Babylon*

2

In high school I was desperate to meet a real homosexual, not like the ones on TV or in movies who were always being arrested or committing suicide. My best friends, Kevin and Michael, were as closeted as I was, so I took it upon myself to see how the other half lived in the shadows. In my sophomore year I called my mother to say I was staying after school to finish an art project. I took a bus to downtown Syracuse and stood across the street from the notorious gay bar called Gotch Carr's. I didn't know what the name meant, but it was the place that kids would crank-call all the time, as in "Is Seymour Butts there?" And a common insult to kids like me was "Going to Gotch Carr's tonight to see your boyfriends, faggot?"

Back at the bus stop I saw my dream man coming toward me down the sidewalk. He stopped and stood with the others waiting for the bus. He had feathered blond hair parted in the middle and a Fu Manchu mustache framing his handsome Nordic face. Tightly fitted across his muscular torso was a spotless white zip-up hoodie with a high waistband. Dark gabardine bell-bottom slacks accentuated his eye-catching crotch and muscular behind. His cream-colored platform shoes made him tower over my frail, youthful frame. A bus arrived, and he got on it. I quickly followed, going through my pockets for change. I took my

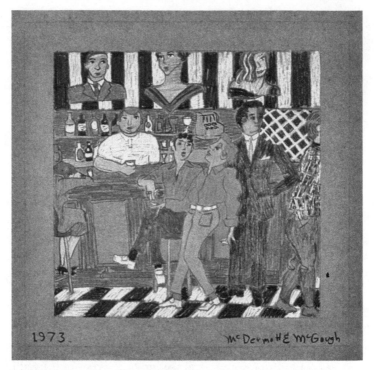

1973.   McDermott E McGough

Gotch Carr's, the Syracuse gay bar I stood across the street from in
hopes of meeting a real homosexual

seat across from him trying to catch his eye through his aviator sunglasses, hoping he'd stop looking out the window and notice me. After
an eternity he called to the bus driver and stood up to exit. I followed
and I found myself in another, unfamiliar suburbia. I don't think I had
ever been this far from my house alone. I could feel my heart beating
with desire. I followed him for a block then summoned the courage
and called out softly, "Hello." He turned and looked at me. I stared
and looked at him against the bright blue sky. It was very quiet. All I
could hear were the birds and the wind through the trees. "Hi," I said.
As he stood looking at me, he asked, "Do you live near here?" I shook
my head. "Then what are you doing here, man?" he asked as he put
his hands on his slim gabardine-covered hips and stared at me. The
heat rose up my face. I wanted him. I lowered my head, paused, and
whispered, "You know."

He tilted his head, asking as he stepped closer toward me, "Know what?" I cleared my throat and repeated much louder, "You know." I knew he knew what I was after. He toyed with me: "I don't know what you're talking about, man. Whatcha looking for?" I stood there in silence waiting for him to take the lead. He just stared at me silently. Humiliated, knowing I couldn't seduce this erotic god before me, I gave up and asked where I could get a bus back to downtown. "Across the street, man," he yawned as he held out his thumb like a hitchhiker and turned and walked away. I crossed the sunny, hot highway and waited for the bus, reprimanding myself for being so foolish and now humiliated as I began my long journey back home to make it in time for dinner.

A month later, I was back downtown. I again stood at the bus stop across the street from Gotch Carr's and waited. I could see men drinking above the curtained brass railing that covered half the window in back of a faded bouquet of paper flowers. I heard a voice addressing me with something about the bus line. I turned to answer a pale blond man with aviator glasses framing his soft blue eyes. On his round face his straight blond hair stuck to his forehead dotted with perspiration. He was wearing a denim leisure suit and carried a plastic shopping bag. He kept talking to me about different subjects and asking me questions. Then it dawned on me that I was with a homosexual; I felt excitement and terror. He said he had a room down the block at the local YMCA where he took naps. Before I knew it, we were in his narrow nap room. After an uneventful act in the nude I lay there planning my exit. I enjoyed the new experience of lying around naked, but I couldn't be late for dinner. I feared my mother might call the school looking for me. She didn't even let me cross the highway till I was thirteen.

Breaking the silence of the room, I asked the inevitable "What do you do?"

"Well . . ." He paused and then declared proudly, "I'm in show business."

"Really?" My interest peaked.

"Oh, yeah," he gleefully answered and turned to face me, leaning on his elbow with his head in his hand, staring at me. I noticed his pale stomach sagged toward the mattress. "Yes, I'm an actor on television." He smiled.

"Oh, wow!" I murmured, thinking how I was with a real, live actor and he's on TV.

"What show are you on?" I asked excitedly, fantasizing about how this pudgy actor would scoop me up and I would live in Hollywood, escorted to film parties, laughing and drinking with my newfound famous actor friends, going to movie premieres, away from this boring suburban world I lived in.

He cleared his throat. "Well, have you ever seen the show *The Enchanted Tree House?*" I could feel the red carpet being pulled out from under me. "Of course," I answered glibly. "I used to watch it. It's a kids' show." My dreams of meeting an actual star immediately fell flat. And the disappointing sex added to my dismay. It was my first time (with an adult), and I thought somehow it would be different, or at least pleasurable.

"Well . . . yes," he stuttered. "Do you know the segment when Cindy and Bobbie"—the stars of the show—"go visit Bumblebee's Backyard?"

"Um, yeah, I know it." I knew this was a bad omen. Now I just wanted to leave.

"Well, I'm Chucky Chipmunk, who dances in Bumblebee's Backyard," he said staring and smiling.

"So much for show business," I thought. After a long pause, and I guess my obvious disappointment, he leaned in flirtatiously, asking, "And what do *you* do?"

By this time, I was annoyed. I dryly stated, "I'm in high school."

His eyes widened as he sat upright on the thin bed. He seemed very much like a frightened child now. "What?!" he shrieked. "Wait, just how old are you?"

"I'll be sixteen in June," I said, pushing his fear to the edge. I was now the spider with the fly.

"What? You're fifteen!" he cried. "Oh, my God . . . Oh, my God!" he whimpered as he put his sweaty round face in his hands. I saw I was in a position of power. For the first time I felt the thrill of it mixed with a feeling of pity for this man sitting on the edge of the bed with his washed-out, pale body. And then I noticed the thin band of gold on his left-hand ring finger. I took pity on him, one closet case to another. "Don't worry," I reassured him. "What do you think I'm going to do—tell my mother?"

I just wanted to go now. I dressed quickly and picked up my book bag. He didn't move at all and just sat there on the bed, staring at the floor. I touched his bare shoulder and said goodbye. I turned, about to open the door. "Thank you," he mumbled. "It was lovely. Thank you."

I bid a last farewell to the stranger who was still sitting on the bed but now lighting a cigarette. He blew smoke up at the ceiling like an old movie star and looked up at me with his big wet eyes and muttered, "I think . . . I mean, I think . . . Well, I think . . . that I'm . . . in love with you." I didn't even know this person and didn't know how to answer him.

"Well, thanks—goodbye," was all I could say as I closed the door.

Back home at dinner my mother asked, "How was the art project?"

"Oh, it didn't go as well as I hoped."

In high school there was one tiny, well-groomed boy in my older brother John's class who was ultra-fey. And no one seemed to bother him. I couldn't believe he got away with being so obviously swishy. And he was a friend of the cool cheerleaders and their handsome jock boyfriends. I'd see him in the hall lounge sitting with the beautiful rich girls while they were brushing their long, silky hair, laughing at some joke and reapplying their pale lip gloss. I'd overhear them talking about winter ski trips at Greek Peak or who was going on the European class trip. And then this little queen ran for president of his class and won!

I could not understand what was wrong with me, why I was not in that group that was laughing, applying lip gloss, and talking about skiing. Why was I a target and not him? Was it because he was from the rich part of town, and rich people were nicer? I didn't understand it. Maybe he had the confidence I did not. He seemed quiet, though. So soft-spoken.

There were other boys in my class who I knew were gay. They didn't have to say anything. It's the way we would look at one another. There always seemed to be a question in our eyes. "Are you one? Could we actually be friends, or more?" But we'd stay away from one another. One male beauty on the track team, whose sister was in my art class, often passed me in the hallway. At those moments, I could feel that he was one of my own. He was even on my school bus, but we never spoke. We never dared. The first day of sophomore year he came on the school bus with his hair bleached such a bright canary blond it was obvious it had been done at home. The boys on the bus went crazy, especially one cruel, ugly kid. He kept yelling out to him "Hey, blondie!" and calling him "Miss Clairol," laughing, trying to get the others to laugh with him. And at the same time, I was glad it wasn't my turn to be mocked. I felt sorry for him. He didn't answer them. He just took it and stared out the window, trying to shut out the forced laughter.

High school was altogether bigger and there were students from outside our particular white suburb. I spent most of my time in the art room learning ceramics, silk screening, and block prints from a nun who encouraged my interests. This is where I made friends with artists and outcasts. The art nun had a quiet young fellow who was her assistant. I called him "Madam Secretary." He looked like he had just stepped out of *The Boys in the Band,* with his tight pants, pointy Beatle boots, big mohair sweater, and sideburns that accentuated his dark, aquiline features. He was a former student, and a friend of his would stop by whom I knew from the school plays when he was a senior and I was a freshman. I could feel the freedom they had after being let out of my high-school prison, and they had the verve of being themselves at last, with a life away from the animals who hunted us in the hallways. I would enter different art contests and usually came in first or second place. My mother clipped a picture from the newspaper of me at a local awards ceremony and put it on our refrigerator door. For the picture

I wore my favorite Marilyn Monroe sweater, plaid bell-bottoms, and saddle shoes.

At home, there was only the dining-room table on which I could make drawings, but no place to paint. There was no attic and the cellar was full from my mother's hoarding. At night I would hitchhike to take life-drawing lessons up the road at a community college. One evening there was a naked man with a beard who was posing. I sat there making figure sketches and grew bored, so to keep myself amused I did an elaborate drawing of his penis and its surrounding dark, full pubic bush. I hitchhiked back home and found my mother again entertaining a few local priests. I put my drawing pad down to shake hands with the guests, but the minute I did so my mother picked it up to show off my drawing abilities to her guests. The page fell open to the crotch drawing. She froze and closed the pad and sharply handed it back to me.

At an early age my mother let me know that she couldn't help me at school and I had to get by and pay attention, but somehow I couldn't. My head was lost in scenarios of good-looking male classmates or the femmes fatales on TV. I did learn how to get others to like and protect me, but that came at a high price. I became the "listener," the "dear friend," the one who'd be the voice of reason. I was the "gal Friday," the best friend, the one who was always available. I perfected the role, which I played seamlessly in high school, but I hated it. I knew my part well. I became the supporting actor, never to rise to the lead role. Then I realized maybe I was a person with talent. And all those years of daydreams and scenarios in my head had a purpose.

I couldn't wait to get out of the house and move to New York. I didn't like the sameness of the suburbs. I wanted the life I saw in the movies. I had a grant to go to either a university in Buffalo or the Fashion Institute of Technology in New York. My oldest sister, Mary Susan, said of FIT, "You don't want to go to that school, it's full of homosexuals." That helped me make my decision. Before I moved to Manhattan, my father had opened a checking account for me with the New York Savings Bank up the highway because they had a branch on

Fifth Avenue. The day before I left home, in early September 1978, I hitchhiked up the highway to a strip mall to make my last bank deposit in Syracuse. The man who picked me up was very friendly and chatty as he massaged his growing crotch. So we took a side route to a dirt road and he blew me in his car.

3

I n late 1978 most of downtown Manhattan, east and west, was dirty
and dangerous. There were piles of rubbish on Seventh Avenue from
FIT's Twenty-Ninth Street dorms to the West Village; Eighth Avenue
was considered unsafe, and we were cautioned by the older students to
stay off it from Fourteenth Street to above the Theater District. And
west of that was also out. The West Village was full of men in leather
outfits or western gear. On any weekend you'd even see a man in a
construction-worker outfit with a tool belt and a hard hat, or someone
who looked like an extra on *Bonanza,* somewhat like a gay version of
the Wild West. The West Side Highway still had the elevated train
tracks above it and was home to the leather bars, places like the Ramrod, the Eagle, Sneakers, and Keller's, among others. Across the highway were collapsing piers where men went to have sex or sunbathe nude.

I loved the West Village, especially in the summer. All the different
types of gays would be out on the street. And there were many protests
for gay rights. There was a character named Rollerena who was a slim
older man in a 1950s party dress, a hat with a veil, lots of sparkling
cheap jewelry, and cat eyeglasses. She spun around on roller skates as
she held a glitter wand with a star on the end, and as she touched passersby on the head she'd squeeze an old brass horn, which made a loud

honk. The neighborhood was full of characters, from the old cocktail queens to leathermen to bohemian artistic types from the past. It was when being a freak was chic.

Times Square was a mess of dirty old theaters that showed horror movies with titles such as *Make Them Die Slowly* and straight porn movies, in front of which were large cutouts of scantily covered women with beehive hairdos. And yet I was thrilled to be living in Manhattan. It was everything I dreamed of and more. I spent my tuition money going to nightclubs after deciding I hated studying illustration and fashion design. The teachers didn't like my drawings. "Too detailed," they'd say. "Just a suggestion with lines!"

One of my drawing teachers was a short Italian man with a mustache. He offered me a job illustrating products for a cosmetics company called Princess Marcella Borghese. I was happy to get the work since I was running out of tuition money. He lived uptown in a doorman building, and his apartment was decorated with wood sectionals covered in gray carpeting and pillows. At the end of one of our workdays he offered me a beer and asked if I wanted to watch some episodes of *I Love Lucy* that he had taped. I was never a fan of Lucy growing up; her hijinks made me nervous.

Lucy was followed by *The Devil in Miss Jones.* "It actually has a good story line," he said. "I mean for porn." I knew I was naive at nineteen, but I quickly declined his sexual advances and soon found I no longer had my job.

At FIT I took up with a handsome boy from New Jersey named Billy Metz. He had a mass of auburn hair that looked like a lion's mane and a natural, beautiful physique.

When we first met I was having a conversation about my idol at the time, Antonio Lopez, the fashion illustrator, whom I read about in *Interview* magazine and whose drawings I saw in the *Times.* Billy interrupted and said he knew him and that if I bought him a bottle of champagne, he'd introduce me. The introduction never happened, unlike the champagne. We were just friends but spent almost every waking hour together. He lived at the Chelsea Hotel with our classmate Curtis, who moved out after he found a large water bug on his pillow when he woke up. "Pretend it's an Egyptian scarab," Billy said, trying to calm him down. Sid Vicious and Nancy Spungen lived down the hall. One night, Curtis had gone to their room to do drugs. That night Sid and Nancy started fighting and Sid hit her on the head. A few weeks later, the police knocked on Billy's door after Nancy was murdered.

One Sunday, drunk and bored, Billy and I started to draw on the hotel walls with crayons, making portraits in frames, or a door. When I went back a week later some other friends came by and drew sliding glass doors showing two bikinied women with beehive hairdos being served drinks by a pool. Soon the walls were covered in Crayola drawings. Billy and I then planned our twenty-first birthday party to take place on Billy's birthday in early July at the Chelsea, sending out the invitations with photo-booth portraits of us for our "21-Gun Salute." On my birthday, June 29, the two of us had drinks at "21," the

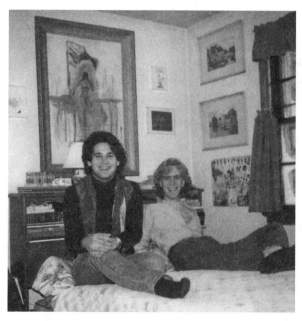

My friend Billy Metz, with Michael Kors

old-guard restaurant on Fifty-Second Street. Billy gave me a key chain from Tiffany's and I gave him three thick-cotton button-down Brooks Brothers shirts in pastels to go with his Lilly Pulitzer jeans or his gold ones from Fiorucci, a trendy store on East Fifty-Ninth Street. I also added a huge bouquet of long-stem yellow roses. The roses thrilled him. He took them out of the box and promenaded down the hallway of the Chelsea making promises as to what he would do as the newly crowned Miss New Jersey.

Our birthday party swiftly filled with our friends, and then the word got out there was a party with a full free bar and our room on the second floor became packed with hustlers and other oddballs who lived at the hotel. We were thrilled that Cookie Mueller, the John Waters actress, even showed up briefly. She eyed the room, said "Hi," and, not knowing anyone, left. I woke the next morning under a pile of garbage bags and wearing a striped minidress. I don't remember how that happened. I looked around the room, littered with our passed-out friends and some naked stranger. On my own I had never really been a drinker or much of a drug taker. I didn't like the hangovers. But if someone was drinking, I drank. And Billy was very persuasive. If this creature of whims was doing drugs, I would, too. I've tried every drug they've made except the romantic opium.

At twenty-one, Billy was a full addict, with his motto being "Drunk before noon." Addicts were adventurous and seemed to be able to do anything, say anything. Being so shy, I was thrilled to go along for the ride. Billy liked to go to the bar on West Tenth Street south of Greenwich Avenue called the Ninth Circle. From 1961 to the early 1970s it had been a steakhouse owned by Mickey Ruskin of Max's Kansas City, frequented by singers and musicians, but in 1971 he sold it to Bobby Krivit, a mobster who, after the Stonewall riots in 1969, turned it into *the* gay bar, with drinks in the front, drugs in the back, and male hustlers playing pool in the cellar.

On my weekly visits to that bar I met Allen Midgette, the Warhol superstar and Andy impersonator, and the poet, critic, and artist Rene Ricard, whom later I would get to know through McDermott and the

East Village art world. This became our usual hangout. Then on to Ty's, Boots & Saddles, Julius', the Ramrod, Sneakers, the Cock Ring (for dancing), or Cars, a "wrinkle room" with a jukebox that played Marlene Dietrich's "Where Have All the Flowers Gone." The drinks were cheap, and we were "chicken." One evening making the rounds we went into a junk shop on Christopher Street and Billy bought an old Chinese figurine-shaped cookie jar that he carried around all evening.

In 1979, I had only been in my apartment on Twenty-Sixth Street and Eighth Avenue a few months when it was robbed, so I moved in with my friend Chuck. Chuck lived with his older boyfriend, Jesse, an astrologer and numerologist, in Jesse's loft on Twenty-Eighth Street and Broadway. Before the robbery, Chuck, who was beautiful and who I had hoped would be my boyfriend, had moved in with me on Twenty-Sixth Street after he took the summer off back home in Memphis. One evening, he and I had gone to see a midnight showing on Eighth Street of the John Waters cult film *Pink Flamingos*. Afterwards we went to Boots & Saddles for a drink, where Chuck left with this guy Jesse and I went home alone to Twenty-Sixth Street. Then Chuck moved in with Jesse to his loft a month later and I was on my own. Once I was robbed I moved in with them; my room had a curtain stapled to the wall as a door. In the loft, I started making a few paintings of abstract imagery influenced by cubism and sixties shop signs, trying to find my style. The neighbor next door, who made boxes for Claes Oldenburg, saw my paintings and told me to look for another profession. I could draw but didn't have the hand or practice for oils. I knew nothing of the contemporary art world except for the big names I learned at school. I did visit museums to look at early-twentieth-century modernism. I was fascinated by Duchamp and Man Ray. I thought that if I could just make paintings, someone would see them, show them, sell them, and it would be easy, just like that. I later found that was not the case.

The summer night of our classmate Michael Kors's nineteenth or twentieth birthday Billy and I ended up at the Ninth Circle in the back garden. Michael was a toothpick of a figure with rings of golden curls above a dewy complexion. I had a funny feeling he'd make it in fashion because he was always so focused, sketching and talking about style, clothes, and the famous. When he first came to school from Long Island, he wore painted-on Sassoon jeans and soft, glove-leather knee-high boots from Italy. He also carried a small square bag he looped around his wrist as his wallet. I'd never seen a man carry what I thought was a purse. We all had our hometown looks before New York changed all that. Mine was longish hair my sister would cut, a few old rags from my father's closet, and a polyester shirt with an illustration on the back of an ashtray with cigarette smoke spelling "Cabaret." Billy disappeared from our table, came back, and pressed tabs of acid to our mouths as he ordered fresh drinks. "Take it—take it!" he badgered us, pushing the tabs against our lips.

Back at the loft, Billy, Michael, and I sat on the floor whispering so as not to wake Chuck and Jesse, while Billy made crank phone calls in the early dawn, saying he was looking for Laura Mars after the Faye Dunaway movie *The Eyes of Laura Mars.* Billy would mix the catchphrases from *Cruising* (starring Al Pacino) and *Laura Mars.* "This is Laura Mars and I'm cruising for a killer," he'd sob softly into the phone. We'd all giggle and hang up after we could hear the other end cursing him. Chuck's boyfriend had a 1940s pink satin ballgown that Billy wore over his clothes as we made the calls. The night ended with Michael and me fishing him out of the fountain in Madison Square Park as he proclaimed, "I am Mahogany! I am Mahogany!" from the Diana Ross movie.

In the late seventies, my classmates from FIT—a clique of the cool fashion queens—and I went to the notorious Studio 54 in an old television studio that Steve Rubell and his partner, Ian Schrager, had opened as a nightclub on Fifty-Fourth Street between Broadway and Eighth Avenue. The busboys wore only satin running shorts and sneakers. Every famous person was quickly ushered through those doors while most people waited behind the velvet ropes. My school friends and I had no trouble being let in because we were young and well dressed. Often a black limousine would show up as the crowd turned and collectively whispered, "Who is it?" The crowd would part as the newly arrived entered. A few would run in with them or be brought in by the door-man. Often, even hours later when you left, there would still be people behind the ropes, spilling out into the street and down the block.

Inside, up in the balcony people leaned over the railing watching the frenzied dancing while behind them people were having "disco naps," either taking drugs or having sex or mostly doing both. The bathrooms were essentially unisex, with people having sex or doing coke in the stalls. Girls were in the boys' room and boys in the girls' room. It didn't matter. It was a mix of the famous and the beautiful and the rich and the poor—as long as you looked good.

At some point in the evening an immense crescent moon would come down surrounded by twinkling lights; a coke spoon followed and went under the man in the moon's nose as light shimmered up from the spoon into his nose. The crowd went wild. Long spinning lights would come down from the ceiling as the music got louder, and at a certain moment in the song colorful cubes of sponge flew out into the crowd as they cheered loudly, picking up the soft gifts. If the Stones' new song "Miss You" or Rod Stewart's "Da Ya Think I'm Sexy?" came on, the crowd would pack the dance floor. One night I was there running around having fun and a young, good-looking fellow my age stopped me and offered me a drink ticket. I didn't have any money to pay for a drink, so I took it. As we sipped our drinks he asked if I wanted to go to the VIP room in the cellar and meet his friend Bob Colacello, the editor of Andy Warhol's *Interview* magazine. "Of course!" I screeched. I knew that's where Liza, Cher, and numerous other celebrities lounged.

"I'm Bob's friend," my host said to the man at the small door. He replied, "The cellar is closed tonight." With a shrug the boy led me up a metal staircase to a room with a freshly made bed in it. The boy started kissing me and trying to remove my clothes. "Wait a minute!" I cried. "Let me put my drink down first!" I placed my half-full drink on the table, and when I turned around he had some pills in his hand. "Here, take this," he said.

"What is it?" I asked.

"It's a Quaalude, man."

"A what?"

"A 'lude, dude. Just take it, baby—you'll feel great!"

I was game, and he was cute and now naked and now helping me shed my outfit. We fell into the bed with the loud thumping of the music below us.

I woke up in the quiet room not knowing where I was or how long I had been there. I looked over at my sleeping companion and remembered.

"Hey." I shook him awake. It was eerily silent. We dressed and stumbled down the metal stairs to the door that opened to the dance floor. The club was vacant. All that was left were the empty glasses and confetti from the night before. The bulbous silver sofas that usually held Halston, Liza, and Warhol were empty. A hush filled the room. "What time is it?" I thought.

"How are we going to get out?" I asked my nameless friend.

"I don't know. Let's try this back door."

We pushed on the bar of the door and in poured the afternoon light. We departed, and I saw that it was three p.m.

"Hey, let's go see Steve," he suggested, meaning one of the owners. "We're friends, he used to invite a bunch of us to his place on Fire Island for fun. I won a jerk-off contest there two weeks ago."

We arrived at Rubell's apartment where the doorman announced us. Rubell was still in bed and his couches matched the ones in his club. The place had the look of an almost-finished hotel room with empty walls.

"Hey, man," Steve said to my friend from his bed.

"This is my friend . . ." He paused.

"Hi, I'm Peter."

"Yeah! Pete, my new friend," the youth said.

He told the story of how we fell asleep at the club to a grumbled laugh from our host. The kid went into the bathroom and I sat there shyly in silence, still feeling the effects of the pill. Luckily Steve made a phone call.

"Oh, yeah, so-and-so was there. . . . No, they never showed. . . . Oh, yeah, it was a great time—well, what I could remember."

The kid came back as Steve was giving out his private number. I saw my bedfellow write it down. Rubell dismissed us and we got on the subway. My one-night stand bit a pill in half and gave me the remainder and said, "This will make you feel better." He then took a pill bottle out of his jacket and emptied a few of the Quaaludes into my hand. "For later, man. I took it from the bathroom," he said, laughing. The train stopped, and he got off. "See ya around, man," he said as he bounced down the platform.

I found a job at a fashion magazine published for the Garment District. It consisted of going around Seventh Avenue to fashion houses sketching their latest collections. The magazine would give an account of the designer's colors and styles for the season. I reported to a stout woman with a perfectly coiffed old-style hairdo who wore a different but similar short-sleeved belted shift every day. She would always be on the phone at her desk, barking out orders. "Tomorrow?!" she'd scream indignantly. "If I wanted it tomorrow I'd have asked for it tomorrow. Have it on my desk by five!" as she slammed down the phone.

Then I saw the coworker who was to escort me to each showroom enter the office. Even at my inexperienced age I could tell she wasn't an ordinary person. She was a weeping willow of a figure, tall and slim, right out of a Norman Parkinson photo from a fifties fashion magazine, or Kay Thompson from the movie *Funny Face*. She would throw her hips forward as she glided across the room. This vision always wore a simple form-fitting shift, ending at midcalf, in plain, soft colors—no patterns. But that simplicity would be decorated around the neck and the arms. The sleeves ended below the elbow, and she always had long gloves and a menagerie of bracelets jingling around her wrists. Her makeup was kabuki white, with a slash of red lips that almost floated off her pale complexion and a pair of choppers any dentist would be proud of. Her dark-eyeliner cat eyes would be hidden behind large green sunglasses that she must have worn for decades. She kept a clutch tucked under her arm and wore a cloche hat and big costume-jewelry earrings and necklace. There was always a long cigarette holder with a smoldering unfiltered Chesterfield butt parked in the side of her mouth that mixed with her heavy perfume. I'd head out with "Slim" and go to the showrooms. Some salespeople, like designer Chester Weinberg's assistant, would silently pull out a rack of the latest hemlines and leave us, while others, like Bill Blass, would have a house model wearing the clothes and serve cookies and coffee which I heartily ate as my lunch. "Slim" wouldn't touch anything except a coffee. As I sat and drew the clothes I was always told to "speed it up," because we had many places to go. She'd look over at my sketch as she pressed a new Chesterfield into her lacquered holder. "Hmm . . . they always seem to look like you," she'd purr.

It was only a part-time job and I needed more income. One morning I called the office to say I was departing to get a full-time job at Trash and Vaudeville on St. Marks Place.

"Typical youth!" my boss shouted. "Do you understand how lucky you are to have this job? And how many people would be happy to be working here?" Now I knew how the people on the other end of the phone felt. As I stammered to explain, she cut me off in mid-sentence. "Never mind, good luck. You'll need it!" she barked, slamming down the phone. My Trash and Vaudeville job only lasted a few months.

4

I t was the heat of the sun on my face that woke me. I didn't open my eyes because in my waking, my head hurt and when I moved to the other side of the damp pillow it started to swim. I heard snoring. I slowly turned my head and opened my eyes. My blurred vision cleared to see a naked, muscular, tattooed man across the room, asleep in another single bed. Between the stranger and me was a small wooden table covered with debris, including an overflowing ashtray, some coins, and a crumpled pack of unfiltered Lucky Strikes. In a bowl of milk, a cockroach was floating on one of the remaining Froot Loops. I closed my eyes and gagged at the sight.

My head was throbbing, and I felt nauseous as I quietly sat up. I remembered I was at a party somewhere the night before and the last thing I could recall was talking to someone who was filling my tumbler with vodka as I downed four pills called Valium (a first for me) that we took from the medicine cabinet of our party host. Or was it at the Hotel Chelsea where Billy lived? I was confused, with no idea how I had arrived at this hellhole.

"Where the fuck am I?" I thought as I looked over the dump I found myself in.

Dirty clothes littered the floor of the small room along with empty liquor bottles and miscellaneous crushed garbage. I wanted to find my clothes since I was naked, too. One of my saddle shoes was near me and I found the other under the bed. Frightened about waking the snoring, muscular, tattooed figure, I quietly gathered my clothes, gingerly stepping over the piles on the floor to make my escape, thinking I'd dress in the hallway. It felt like the room was spinning. I tiptoed to the exit, silently turned the many locks, and slowly opened the door. As it made a loud, horror-house squeak, I held my breath and clenched my jaw.

"Where are you going?" a deep, crackled voice addressed me. I let out a quivering sigh as I turned toward the stranger. "Oh . . . hi." I was still naked with my clothes and shoes tightly held to my aching chest. "Sit down," he ordered. Like the inexperienced youth I was, I did what I was told. "Name's Don," he coughed out. All I could answer was "Peter." He yawned and stretched as he stood in his muscular, tattooed magnificence, lighting a crumpled cigarette with a matchbook that read "The Haymarket," a notorious rough-trade hustler bar in Times Square. He shook his head and scratched his skull through his wavy brown hair, which hung past his wide, strapping shoulders.

"Excuse me. Um . . . how did I get here?" I muttered. I was still holding on to my clothes at the end of his bed, shivering.

"Oh, yeah," he laughed. "I found you passed out in the gutter last night and I threw you over my shoulders and brought you home." I thought of the school jingle "When I see trash I pick it up." He kept on mumbling through his yawns about hanging out at Port Authority waiting for the young ones getting off the bus and moving to the city, but I wasn't really listening. I was cold, and I just wanted to get out of there. And I didn't want to throw up in the room.

"I have to go now," I interrupted.

As I stood up he said, "You're not going anywhere just yet, sweet cheeks," and pushed the door closed.

On the street, I found myself in the bright morning of an empty Times Square: the old Forty-Second Street of dirty porno houses where men slept or had sex with each other, decrepit peep shows, and prostitutes of both sexes. In the punishing light I saw how soiled my clothes were from the gutter. I scoured my pockets and found my old sunglasses to dim the intense light of a cloudless sky. I pulled together some crumpled bills and bought a huge tumbler of Coca-Cola and downed it to revive my ill state. "This can't be my life," I cried as I walked downtown. "I didn't move to New York to be a bar hag." And I was just raped. My clothes stank of cigarette smoke and the gutter. I started to cry, thinking of my good Christian parents and of how horrified they'd be. Plus, my father was now sick with cancer. They hadn't wanted me to attend school in New York City. When I moved to Manhattan, my mother sewed a cloth pouch for me to keep my money in and had me safety-pin it to my underpants. I had no direction except following others to bars and clubs, downing drinks and doing drugs. I felt like I was slowly drowning. I looked up at the bright sky and whispered hoarsely, "Please, somebody, help me."

I was spending time again at my usual hangout, the Ninth Circle. One evening as I was wondering what I was doing with my life, drowning my sorrows in a vodka and making Olympic-flag rings with my wet glass, I looked up from the bar to see two tall, slim youths walking toward me. They had a casual but distinct 1930s Manhattan look and stood out from the jeans-and-T-shirt crowd, especially the one who looked like the actor Basil Rathbone. I guess I was staring when they were passing my table because the other one said, "Heeeellooooooo, I'm Jeffrey," in a long-drawn-out introduction, flashing a toothy grin. The Basil Rathbone look-alike extended his hand. "I'm Daniel," he said. I noticed his pencil-thin mustache and manicured nails. And he was wearing a tie for a belt, like Fred Astaire.

They sat in the empty chairs at my table and we chatted. They were buying, so I had more drinks. I explained my dilemma: my roommate Chuck's "clone" boyfriend, Jesse, had asked me to move out of their loft on Twenty-Eighth Street. Jeffrey interrupted and said he was looking for a roommate. He had just thrown out two people who over-stayed, and his place was ten minutes away, off Bleecker Street. I was a bit shocked by his swift offer, but being desperate, I accepted. The next week, with my suitcase, some Andrews Sisters and David Bowie records, and my art portfolio, I moved into his ground-floor apartment.

He had a small, one-bedroom apartment with windows on the street decorated in a 1930s style with chrome-and-leather office furni-ture and green cubist wallpaper. The very dark bedroom in the back was packed with boxes and clothing racks full of clothes from many different decades, including shimmering gowns, wool suits, and flow-ered Hawaiian shirts. Jeffrey would sell them on West Broadway on the weekends. I didn't see a bed in sight. When it was time for bed, Jeffrey pulled out of the heap in the back a thin, dirty piece of foam, mismatched sheets, and two flat old pillows.

"Well, it ain't the Ritz," he giggled.

What did I care? I was desperate and tired. In my naiveté I lay down on the grimy-sheeted foam. During the night I had to push him off me a couple of times as he nestled his head on my shoulder.

Jeffrey would take me around Manhattan and show me the fading past of the city. In Times Square there was the shoe store I. Miller, which had four stone statues that sat in gold tile arches of Ethel Bar-rymore, Marilyn Miller, Mary Pickford, and Rosa Ponselle, carved by Alexander Stirling Calder, the sculptor's father, who also did the two George Washington sculptures on the east and west piers of the Washington Square Park Arch. Above was a carved slogan, "The Show Folks Shoe Shop Dedicated to Beauty in Footwear." The façade is still there buried under large burger advertisements. Close by I was shown an old "ten cents a dance" club down a flight of stairs that had two large circular murals of flappers dancing, painted in a primitive style.

When Jeffrey took me to the revival-house cinema the Thalia, on the Upper West Side, to see a Bette Davis and Joan Crawford double feature, I was taken aback by the mostly male audience laughing and catcalling as the drama unfolded. This was my first real introduction to camp.

Every morning when Jeffrey turned on the old stove, ten cockroaches of different sizes ran out. I was used to roaches on Twenty-Eighth Street with Chuck, but this looked like a mass exodus. Jeffrey served the coffee in a modernist tea set and put the bagels on Fiestaware plates. Between our chatter and the crooner on a record player we were getting to know each other. I found him to be quite funny and sweet. But I was hoping he didn't have designs on me. Among the colorful breakfast dishes was a silver-framed photo of a young man staring out at me with pomaded hair parted down the middle, wearing Harold Lloyd round glasses and an artistic floppy cravat engulfed by a fur-lapeled coat. "Who's that?" I asked curiously.

"Oh, that's David McDermott—he's crazy!" He frowned. "I had to throw him and his boyfriend, Walter, out. They were supposed to stay one night, and they stayed over a month!" He went on ranting, and I was sorry I asked. Then he abruptly changed the subject back to

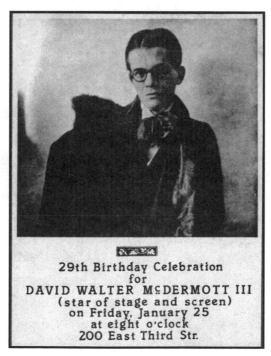

29th Birthday Celebration
for
DAVID WALTER McDERMOTT III
(star of stage and screen)
on Friday, January 25
at eight o'clock
200 East Third Str.

The photo of McD I saw on the table at Jeffrey's

himself and showed me some beautiful photographs I thought were old images of two women in drop-waist dresses standing in front of a 1930s mirrored dresser. But Jeffrey said that he had taken them and started lecturing me about his work. As he lifted his coffee cup to his lips he stared at me, batting his long lashes and letting out a long sigh. "Ahmmmm. . . . But you're very sweet."

"Oh, no," I thought. "There's going to be tears—and not mine."

"Peter, you have to go see David McDermott perform! He reminds me so much of you, and he's funny just like you," said Jody Morlock, a pint-sized girl with a face like a fifties Avedon model. A year earlier Jody tried to pick me up at Studio 54. Sitting on the steps to the balcony, she had asked me above the din of the disco music if I liked boys or girls. I pointed to my pink suit and said, "Guess."

Jody went on to tell me about the "New Wave Vaudeville" at Irving Plaza, an old Polish social hall just above Fourteenth Street. The show had many different acts, from a stripper named Lady Bug with hand puppets (she later made it to *The Gong Show*) to rock-and-roll performances. I had read about Klaus Nomi, at the start of the show, in Glenn O'Brien's column in *Interview*. He was a pale German pastry chef who brought to mind Marlene Dietrich Meets Dracula from Outer Space. He wore a clear plastic cape and a skintight space suit, as he sang in falsetto an aria from the opera *Samson et Dalila* to canned music while smoke rose around him. At each performance McDermott had to explain to the audience that the accompaniment was recorded but the singing was live. Nomi always received an uproarious standing ovation at the end. That weekend I went by myself to see my doppelgänger sing and dance. McDermott opened the show with a King Tut number, singing as he came in carried by scantily dressed slave boys:

> *Pharaoh*
> *They call me Pharaoh*
> *Being a god could go straight to my head*

Pharaoh
They call me Pharaoh
Just look me up in the Book of the Dead
All the hieroglyphics
Say that I'm terrific
That's why I'm the King of the Nile.

King Tut wore a large Egyptian-style necklace made of Chiclets gum. Throughout the night he introduced each act wearing full-dress tails, with a sly comment or a cornball joke. He was a mixture of the comedian Eddie Cantor and Alfalfa from *The Little Rascals*. He knew how to control the crowd, make them laugh or pay attention, and I could see how comfortable he was onstage. There were lots of bon mots and witty repartee before each act. Lady Bug, the stripper, with an ostrich puppet who peeled her clothes off, had just finished. Men in suits and sunglasses with fake foam guitars danced and acted to rock music as the foam guitars bobbed. "Now, wasn't that wonderful?" McDermott would taunt. "So much talent and practice went into it. Wasn't that lovely?" He'd facetiously laud them and introduce another act in a voice that mimicked an old-time radio announcer. He had my attention. He sparkled every time he came on. The boring acts were the time to refresh one's drink. Then he came out and did a striptease, singing "A Pretty Girl Is Just Like a Pretty Boy," taking off all his clothes down to a one-piece undergarment with garters holding up his socks. The last thing he removed was his fake front tooth.

In the crowd after the show I spotted him smiling, surrounded by admirers. I shyly went up to him when the others departed. "Hello," I shouted over the music. "I'm Peter, Jeffrey's new roommate."

Up close I saw how impeccably dressed he was. He wore a full-dress tail suit with a stiff-starched bright white bib shirtfront with studs, a detachable wing collar with a perfectly tied piqué white bow, and black patent-leather dancing pumps, and his lacquered hair, parted in the middle, was as shiny as his shoes. I couldn't tell his age. He seemed part child, part old man. His comical face was somewhere between fourteen and forty. He had big brown cow eyes, a Bob Hope ski-jump nose, and a mile-wide Hollywood smile. His missing front tooth added to the comical effect. Standing next to him was a smaller, cuter version of him in a 1920s lounge suit. They both stared at me, then at each other, then back at me.

"Oh, look, Walter," David said snidely, "it's Jeffrey's new roommate, Peter," his cinematic smile pinned across his face. "Oh, really," hissed Walter. "How nice."

"Well, goodbye," David waved, dismissing me as they turned and disappeared into the crowd, laughing. Somewhat embarrassed, I was left standing there with my now warm drink and, not knowing anyone, departed.

In the late 1970s and early '80s there were young people who seemingly created a whole persona with an outfit; some looked like versions of Mamie Van Doren or the more obvious Marilyn Monroe in a 1950s party dress; there were male youths dressed in slim-fitting sharkskin suits or baggy 1940s pinstripes from the same thrift stores homeless men on the Bowery used. The youths in the East Village were influenced by the look of French New Wave cinema (Jean-Paul Belmondo) or fifties rockabilly coolness or the kinetic look of punk. This was all before the next generation of suburban kids could watch MTV and get fashion tips. You may not have had a dime, but you could look like a million dollars.

I was walking down Delancey Street one afternoon among the crowds of Polish and Latino locals. Through the mob I saw Blondie singer Deborah Harry and her drummer, Clem Burke, draped in black and wearing dark shades. You have to remember that most men were still wearing gabardine slacks and had feathered hair. I had a new job, which lasted about a year, in an Iranian suit store on Fifty-Seventh Street between Madison and Park, and when the shah of Iran was overthrown in 1979 the framed photograph of him that hung over the office desk was immediately tossed into a garbage can. I worked with a fellow named Richie, a good-looking Jewish guy from Long Island with a thick accent who wore gabardine slacks and had feathered hair.

His Afghan hound was named Champagne. When he bought Blondie's latest album his friends asked him if he was "going punk." To me Debbie and Clem stood out like giants among the masses. Not only because of their fame but their attitude of cool. I stopped and watched them as they passed. They were as oblivious to the crowd as the crowd was to them. To my twenty-one-year-old eyes they were giants.

About two weeks later a friend of Jeffrey's, Paul Bridgewater, popped his head into the open front window and invited Jeffrey to his party that coming Friday. "And bring your little friend," he coyly suggested. That Friday I again wore my favorite outfit: a pale-pink 1950s linen suit, a Hawaiian shirt with a postcard pattern, and my new saddle shoes. The very elderly shoe salesman in the Midtown shop warned me, "Get 'em before the college kids buy 'em all!" My hair was freshly cut ("Long on the top, short on the sides") at Astor Barber for five dollars. We took a taxi over to the East Village to Paul's apartment on East Third Street at Avenue A. It was decorated in shades of black, white, and gray, furnished sparsely with a few pieces of fifties furniture and vintage black-and-white photographs of flowers hanging on the walls. It reminded me of a room from Peter Bogdanovich's film *The Last Picture Show*. The party was full of people with quirky looks: there was an elderly woman (dressed in black) with a shaved head and a dead sardine hanging from one ear. I also met the inventor of the "pink mink." The only person I knew was my roommate, who quickly disappeared into the crowded room.

I saw a Judy Garland imitator in a glittering dress, who on closer inspection turned out to be Walter Fleming, the person with David at the "New Wave Vaudeville" show. He was dancing with a thin man in a black turtleneck and sunglasses who towered over him. Walter had an empty glass in one hand, and looped around the other wrist was a plastic alligator on a rubber band that would bounce up and down as he shimmied. He later told me it was his purse. I reintroduced myself. "Oh, yeah, sure!" Walter yelled over the music. "Come on," beckoning me to join their dance. "We're having a go-go. Get with it!" He then pointed to his partner as they swerved to the beat.

"This is . . . uh . . ." Walter pointed.

"Ted," the tall one shouted.

"Right!" Walter laughed, "Ted! Old friends," as he shook his head and shrugged.

"Hey," he continued, as he feigned a Southern-belle accent, "would you be a doll and get me a refill?" He thrust the warm glass into my hands. "I'm spittin' cotton, honey. And come right back, sugar." As I turned to find the bar, he screamed out, "Vodka! And don't be stingy, baby!" I was relieved he was so funny and friendly.

I crossed the room toward a messy table with different kinds of liquor bottles and bowls full of crumbs. I found a somewhat clean glass for myself and filled that and Walter's with vodka and a few small cubes from a pool in a metal ice bucket. On my way back, I spotted David sitting alone on a boomerang-shaped sofa. Nervously I reintroduced myself, "Hi, David." He looked up at me. He was also in a dress, though not as colorful as Walter's. He wore a subdued gray drop-waist frock, opaque white hose, and sensible, low-heeled suede shoes. His red hair was without pomade and swept across his forehead. I could see how red it was without the paste. Draped over his shoulders hung a 1940s mink jacket.

"I'm Peter," I shouted a bit nervously. "I met you after your show two weeks ago. I'm Jeffrey's roommate." He stared up at me, seemingly trying to remember.

"Oh, yes," he said blankly. "Here, come sit next to me." He patted the sofa.

To break the ice I blurted, "You look nice."

"Oh, well, you don't say," he said with a theatrical "yuk-yuk" kind of laugh. As he held out his hand he let his wrist go limp. Abruptly Walter interrupted with two fresh drinks, "Hey! What happened? Come on!" He gave me an intense stare. I didn't know what to expect. "I ran into David," I mildly squeaked.

"I see that. What about the go-go? I was waiting for my drink!" he snapped. "Here," he shoved a glass in my direction spilling the liquid onto David's dress. "Walter!" David shrieked, "Cut it out!" as he started to blot the dress with a plaid handkerchief that was tucked into his dress. I could tell they had been fighting from their chilly distance.

"Oh, you're all right," Walter moaned.

"He's drunk," David turned and whispered to me.

Walter just feigned a laugh and looked at me. "Well?" I felt I was between two comets. I was tongue-tied. "The go-go?" he yelled.

I left the party late, in tow with Jeffrey and a tipsy Walter. His makeup had smeared from the dancing, and I saw a keychain dangling out of his rubber alligator's mouth. On the street in the cool morning air I asked about David's whereabouts.

"Who cares about him? He's a drag," he slurred. "But you're not— you're fun. I'm gonna have a dinner party for you!" He pointed at me and belched, "Excuse me . . . Next week!" His squinting eyes looked over at Jeffrey. "Oh . . . I guess *you* can come, too."

"I live just at that corner," he sang, pointing down the street, "right above Wing Ding Chicken." I looked in the pointed direction at the ghostly figures milling about under the dim streetlights.

"See ya," he waved with his back to us as he swayed into the darkness.

A week later, on the night of the dinner party, I headed east toward Avenue B and Third Street where the given address was "right above Wing Ding Chicken." I was living off Bleecker Street in Greenwich Village, the birthplace of folk music. A few cafés and bars were still in business where Joan Baez and Bob Dylan had their starts.

Not understanding lower Manhattan, east or west, and having a bad sense of direction, I crossed a virtually empty Washington Square Park. Still going the wrong way, I came to Tompkins Square Park on Avenue A. It looked like a shantytown of cardboard boxes and blue pieces of plastic as tents. I had heard how dangerous "Alphabet City" was, especially after sundown. Avenue A was "A-okay," Avenue B was "B-ware," Avenue C was "C you later," and Avenue D was "Do not enter." I couldn't believe how run-down this part of town was. I didn't know what to expect. Finally, as I walked closer to Avenue B and Third Street it became very crowded, but it also became darker, and not just because the night was upon me. The corner had the effect of an odd

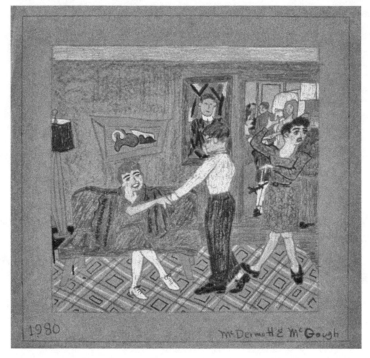

1980

I am meeting David McDermott on the sofa at Paul Bridgewater's apartment; Walter is dancing on the right.

street fair minus the booths. Dubious-looking characters milled about on the sidewalk and into the street, not bothered by passing or crawling cars. The street and sidewalk there knew no separation. People of all ages were outside, sitting on cars and stoops or hanging out windows. A few were passed out on the sidewalk. Loud Latino music was blasting out a window somewhere. Men shouted out into the crowd names of drugs. "Shrooms, sens!" screamed one man for mushrooms and pot. "Black Parrot, Black Parrot!" cried another for heroin.

On the corner I spied a tiny withered woman in a zip-up house-dress and worn slippers standing in front of a grocery cart from Key Foods. In her trolley was a small fire she tended as she cooked skewered meat to sell to the men on the street. I cringed at her burnt offerings. "Where the fuck am I?" I nervously asked myself. It was now night and the street lamps started blinking on. Everything seemed to move in a decelerated way as I took in the street of buyers and sellers. Then out of nowhere a man's face was in front of me. "Hey, white boy. What are you looking for? I can hook you up." His face was inches from mine. I noticed a deep scar down his chin and a tattooed tear under one eye. His black-linear homemade tattoos of Jesus and Mary stood out on his muscular bare chest. Unlike today, one was afraid of tattooed people.

I let out a whimper. "No, I'm just looking for my friend."

"You lookin' for a friend, baby?" he whispered, grinning as he touched my arm.

"Uh . . . no," I stammered. "I'm looking for my friend Walter."

Then, suddenly, out of the noise of the dark, busy street I heard my name being called: "Peter . . . PEETER!"

I sharply turned toward the voice and saw Walter at a window, waving to me from the floor above the infamous sign reading "Wing Ding Chicken" in bold red letters. He was pointing to a door below him. I bolted from the scruffy salesman, weaving my way through the crowd to the door. I heard the man laughing behind me. "What's the hurry, baby?" The door opened and there stood Walter in a crisp starched apron.

"Hi, come on up!" With a concerned look he asked, "Are you all right?"

I was gasping, "Well . . . I mean . . . I . . . uh . . . all those people!"

He looked out at the crowded street. "Meh—they're harmless."

We climbed up a dark slum staircase and entered into another realm very different from the chaos below. As Walter opened the door, I could see a large room with a dining table set in period china and silverware. The whole apartment looked as if I'd entered a silent-movie set. A 1920s sofa and two easy chairs filled the room behind the table. A fringed lampshade hovered over the sofa, and cheap vintage paintings and prints, hung with silk cords, covered the papered walls. I peeked into one of the two period bedrooms to see a large wooden bed and matching dresser. Walter went over to a crank Victrola and put the needle on a 78 rpm record. A male crooner sang in syncopated jazz: "You, you're driving me crazy." Everything was from the past, even the intact period kitchen. There were no modern elements, neither television nor radio. Everything down to an ashtray was from the twenties.

Walter handed me a martini. I heard Jeffrey call up from the street below as Walter threw the key to him out the window. "I ain't climbing the stairs again for *her*," he mumbled.

Jeffrey arrived perfectly outfitted in a 1930s suit but carrying the saddest bouquet. He handed the wilting flowers to Walter as he tilted his head at me batting his eyelashes and smiling. "Heeeelllooo," he sang. I quickly downed my drink.

"Oh . . . that was fast! Good. Time for another." Walter gleefully grabbed my glass.

"Where's David?" I asked.

"Oh, we broke up. He's crazy! Don't get me wrong, he's great—but crazy. I couldn't take it. He's staying with Bradley and Kristian on the Bowery." I was sorry he wasn't there.

A slender, rarefied French queen, Roland Nivelais, who rented the other bedroom, joined us for dinner. Still in his apron, Walter served us a dish of chicken and prunes swimming in a broth. It looked like he threw some cut grass on top of it. He caught me staring at my meal. "Eat. You'll love it. I got the recipe out of *Gourmet* magazine."

"And we're switching to champoozel," he announced as he placed a flute in front of my dish.

Walter and I became good friends. He had a warm, funny personality and an interesting past before McD. He was a deejay at Club 82, an old drag bar off Second Avenue where the glitter rock stars, like the New York Dolls, played, and as a deejay he went by the name "Little Walter." When he was a teenager he worked at Max's Kansas City as a busboy, and before that he would sneak out of his suburban bedroom window in Yonkers in a satin bell-bottom suit he made to take the train in to see the Dolls or Wayne/Jayne County and other rising glitter-rock singers. He knew all the bands and the groupies like Sable Starr, one of the best-known groupies during the glam-rock period, who reportedly slept with Jagger, Bowie, Iggy Pop, and others. He loved disco and funk music and had a huge collection of vinyl records (which McD later gave to sax player James Chance) and hung around the same downtown scene as David. Walter met David through a group of gays who all dressed in 1930s style. Walter explained to me he met McD on the street one day and David had no place to live and was wandering around homeless. Walter invited him to live in his 1920s studio apartment, which faced an air-shaft in a doorman building on Second Avenue. He had thought he would stay only a few nights, but they soon became a couple. I listened in amusement to his stories of how McD would use Walter's expensive Erno Laszlo face soap to wash his feet. Or how they moved to Miami and got jobs in a big Spanish-style mansion. Their employer was a bachelor octogenarian whose mother supposedly owned the cursed Hope Diamond. ("He looked like a living skull," David told me later.) After being shown all morning how to open and close the shades during the day and how to serve a frozen dinner with the correct wineglasses and silverware taken from a large safe, they were dismissed and sent to their quarters. That evening they were locked in their bedroom. After only one night of servitude, as soon as the bedroom door was unlocked in the morning, they escaped back to Manhattan. After a while of getting to know David and Walter in their on-again, off-again relationship, Walter called me to meet him. He informed me that he was taking a job in Florida at a fashion company and closing up the Avenue B apartment and trucking all the contents to his and David's country home, "Wardle House," in Hudson, New York. He was going to send for David after he settled.

"I thought you two broke it off for good?" I asked.

"Meh—who knows? Anyway, David will be alone, so I want you to look out for him. He'll be staying with Bradley and Kristian for a few weeks."

"Oh . . . Okay," I said, not knowing what was in store for me.

5

I n 1979, through Jody Morlock's English boyfriend, Sean Cassette, who was a deejay, I had been hired to help paint a new nightclub called Danceteria. It was on Thirty-Seventh Street near a dangerous part of Eighth Avenue. Danceteria was the brainchild of a Stonewall riot alumnus/Yippie/rock promoter/actor/leftie named Jim Fouratt and his German partner in crime, Rudolf Pieper.

After the place was painted in the latest New Age design, I was then hired as a busboy, picking up bottles, mopping up vomit and blood spills along with other busboys like Keith Haring, David Wojnarowicz (who took me to see a dancing chicken in Chinatown), and fireman Steve Buscemi. Zoe Leonard was the coat-check girl. A sweet, muscular manager named Sunshine, wearing a large Afro and a matching mesh top and bell-bottoms, showed me the correct way to mop a floor. A lot of Brooklyn look-alikes right out of *Goodfellas,* sporting white shoes and leisure suits, were there every afternoon with numerous gold chains around their necks and pinky rings, milling about and whispering before the club opened. One fellow had a toupee that kept getting longer then shorter each week. We'd all gossip and stare when he came with a longer one, then still longer, then back to short. But we didn't mess with those guys because they carried weapons.

With Walter gone, David's attention was solely on me and he courted me throughout the summer. After crying about how I hated my job as a busboy to Chuck, who was now a club bartender, he spoke with a manager to get me a job selling drink tickets, a tricky way of selling booze without a license. I heard that Chuck had told him, "Peter's too fragile to clean up the messes, and upset about his wardrobe being ruined." I was embarrassed, but thrilled to be able to sit all night in a booth from which I could see all the many bands that played, like the Go-Go's or Devo. McDermott would come to the nightclub around four or five a.m. all washed and dressed in a vintage suit, tie, and hat; he usually went to bed at eight p.m. and then headed out when most clubgoers were totally high or exhausted. He'd sit by my booth and get free orange juice. Groovy downtowners didn't pay for entry or drinks. Over the noise he'd shout, "How can they stand this music? It's horrible!—Well, they're not playing the music I like!"—meaning 1920s dance music. He'd wait till I was finished at eight a.m. and I'd take him to breakfast since he never seemed to have a dime. He had just woken up a few hours before and was chatty and energetic, while I, in the meantime, was worn out after the long hours and doing hits of cocaine to stay awake past dawn. Then he'd walk me home to my dirty foam mattress.

To Jeffrey's chagrin David was there every day when I woke up and opened the shade, sitting on the sidewalk right outside the street window. Of course, I'd invite him in for coffee. We'd sit and chat or I'd take some Polaroids of him. We chatted about the night before or some grand idea he had about the past and the hideousness of the present and the horror of things to come. He'd spout ideas of how he didn't want to be living in the present with what he'd call all the "T-shirt tagalongs." "And I *hate* printed T shirts!" he'd say. "It's like wearing a sandwich board. Shouldn't people get paid for advertising someone else's product?"

Once in conversation his tone became serious. "You know, Peter, 1928 is coming back, and I'm ready." He looked ready. "And the future has been canceled! We're all marching off a cliff to the future. For what?

Hideousness, that's what! I've seen the future and I'm not going! And I'm serious! Very serious! The future is finished!" he'd state as his voice escalated. I was convinced he really believed it. David would tell me stories about how he loved to throw parties and how he had met Michael O'Donoghue and other writers from *Saturday Night Live.* He told me about his art salon on the Upper West Side in the early 1970s where he had entertained the likes of the painter Alice Neel (she wanted David to sit for a portrait, but he never did), who had her first retrospective in 1974 at the age of seventy-four at the Whitney Museum; she complained to David that it took too long for it to happen. David's mother was also at the opening, and she went up to a man and asked him why he was wearing a necklace of plastic army men. He turned out to be the correspondence artist Ray Johnson.

Jeffrey warned me, "Peter, I hope you know that David McDermott is crazy!" David had a reputation that preceded him all over town. Even Chuck asked, "Why do you pick such crazy people to be around?" I guess he was speaking about Billy, too. McD told me that once when he was at a Korean grocery, the store clerk showed him some oranges and he believed she was telling him the secrets of the universe. I did not realize he was actually serious. At that point, I found him fascinating and worldly.

There was a striking young woman with wild hair tied in a scarf at Danceteria who hung out near the deejay booth dancing with a group of gay youths. "Who's that?" I asked a bartender. "Oh, her. She goes by the name Madonna," he said, rolling his eyes. Later, she was on the cover of a downtown magazine called *Island,* and the queens were all gushy about her and how she was going to become a big star, that she dated Jean-Michel Basquiat and befriended Keith Haring. She was a definite part of downtown.

When I started selling drink tickets, the minimum wage was $3.10, and I worked eight p.m. till eight a.m. four nights a week. My ticket booth was right next to the bar, and I noticed the drink tickets I just sold were in a large bucket. One night I picked up a handful and resold them in my booth. It padded my low salary, so I kept going back to the bucket. Once one starts a life of crime it's difficult to stop. So, more and more trips to say hello to the very busy bartenders led to another handful. Then one of the bartenders caught me. I thought I'd be sacked but instead he wanted in. Now I didn't have to leave my booth. Then another bartender found out and *he* wanted in. "Okay," I whispered, "but that's it, no one else." Soon, I was supporting David. And then Walter had a new job in a fashion store called All That Glitters. McD suggested they change the name to Al Glitz and Sons, Established 1932.

One evening Danceteria had a private party for the Rolling Stones' new album. It was so VIP that the club was empty, and the Stones looked bored. Outside was a mob of kids that wanted to get in, including McDermott. When the doorman, who knew most of the people, kept apologizing that he was just obeying orders, McD became so enraged he screamed, "If you don't let me and this whole group of downtown society in, I will use all my influence to make Mick Jagger into the next Wayne Newton!" I guess it worked because the doorman opened the velvet rope and in poured the mob of downtown society.

One day David called and asked me to lunch at the Elephant & Castle restaurant close by. "My treat," he offered.

"Give me ten minutes," I said.

I went through the suitcase I was still living out of to find an outfit. I put on a pair of black seersucker trousers and a cowboy shirt with an embroidered square-dancer on it, raked my hair down, and bolted to the restaurant.

McD arrived late, but perfectly dressed in a light suit, yellow cotton gloves, a straw boater hat, and a bamboo walking stick—all tied together with the most perfectly fussed polka-dot bow tie. The whole restaurant turned to stare at his arrival. This apparition mesmerized me. I had never seen anyone dressed so perfectly stepping out of the past. I was only twenty-one, and he fawned over me in a way I had never experienced. As we sat in the window we discussed such strange subjects as the English way of eating vs. the American, clothing, and etiquette. There was no small talk or gossip with McD. He wanted me to understand how serious he was in his conviction of stopping time and living in "another dimension." The modern world held no interest for him. It bored him, and he found it cheap and vulgar.

"You know, Peter, I've seen the past. I've smelled it! I've broken into abandoned houses where everything was still there, down to the Indian-head pennies on the dresser. All the clothes were still hanging in the closet. I could feel the people who once lived there." Then he explained how he was arrested and jailed for breaking and entering. "Now, I wasn't stealing!" he defended himself. "Well, since we're on the subject," he continued, "I was arrested for grand larceny, too. Just so you know. And," he sighed, "a few other times. But nothing too serious."

I had never met a jailbird before. I knew I had met a very strange person indeed, but he was definitely an original thinker. At least he didn't talk about people from outer space. (Not yet—that came later.) He also told me, "Peter, you know I'm a genius." I'd never heard anyone say that, except for Truman Capote on some TV show.

He didn't just read a book or see a film and recount it. He had a theory about what was behind the story or how it worked with history—his favorite subject. He could remember dates, names, geography, and what countries merged or were taken over. He knew the history of the Jews so well he could have taught it. He read almost every book on Jewish history. He'd go on about the original Jews of King David, then those who had converted to Judaism in the Middle Ages or from the eighteenth century. It all fascinated him. He told me the name McDermott was an adopted one and that his birth father was a Yugoslavian Jew who left his mother in Hollywood, three weeks after he was born. The last they heard of him was that he was living in Las Vegas. He also told me his birth father was an interpreter at the UN and spoke many languages. When he was growing up, he asked his grandmother if it was true that his father was Jewish. She replied,

"Of course he was. He had the map of Jerusalem written all over his face." His mother, Vivian, moved back to New Jersey to live with her mother and four-week-old baby, David. Vivian would never talk about her past relationship with his father. She would say to David, "Spare me the misery of recounting my unhappiness."

"And what about you?" He abruptly changed the subject as he devoured sugar cubes from a bowl on the table. I started my story of an ordinary childhood in upstate New York in a vast white suburban neighborhood and how boring I found living there. He obviously grew bored with the blandness of my story because he swiftly switched it back to himself. He knew how to draw me in with a story.

He spoke more of his southern grandmother, Adele, aka Nana, whose mother put her in an orphanage when she was a young girl. Nana's mother said she couldn't take care of so many children. Nana's younger sisters, Edele and Odele, were toddlers at the time. An older boy in the institution showed little Adele what grass and leaves to eat in the forest since they didn't feed them much at the orphanage. She then met a thirty-five-year-old farmer with red hair: "His name was King, and he bought me a Coke-Cola." Adele was introduced to the farmer's mother who asked her son, "Where'd ya get this kid?" When he heard this story, the young David asked Nana, "Didn't you think his mother was stupid?" Nana replied, "Well, she was a lot smarter than I was!" Soon the fourteen-year-old Adele was with child. When she went back to her mother's house with a baby—Vivian—Adele's mother asked, "Where's your man?" "It ain't what I thought it would be," was all she could muster.

As we left the restaurant near dusk, I thought I had found a nice friend, someone to talk to. Little did I know how this person would shape my life.

At this time, David was living at the end of the Bowery on Grand Street in a small corner room with large windows. One set of windows looked out onto the stately Bowery Savings Bank. The other set looked out onto a men's shelter/hotel where, in each room, you could see a man reclining on a single bed. David's room was sparely furnished with a

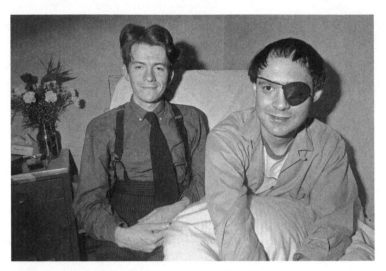

David visiting Bradley Field, a star of the New York punk scene, in the hospital

Victorian single brass bed, a painted dresser, one chair, and a sink that caught the water in a plastic bucket underneath.

His landlords and friends Kristian Hoffman and Bradley Field were ensconced in the downtown punk scene of Max's Kansas City and CBGB, with such punk luminaries passing through as Lydia Lunch, the Cramps, James Chance, and others. Kristian also wrote songs for David when he performed in the "New Wave Vaudeville" show.

The apartment of Bradley and Kristian was dominated by Kristian's collection of Donny and Marie dolls, Kiss dolls, and Victorian devil figurines, mixed with all sorts of objects too many to list. I told Kristian I used to go see his band the Mumps at Max's.

McDermott had been involved in the downtown world of the East Village of the mid-1970s. In the early 70s, when he was living on the Upper West Side, McD swallowed an economy-size bottle of aspirin, was found by a neighbor stumbling on the street in a nightshirt, and then checked himself into the psych ward at Bellevue where a nurse he became friendly with suggested he check himself out, because after three days they can keep you up to six months for observation. This had all been triggered by Kristian's rejection of him. Afterwards he came out to his parents. They sent him to a shrink. McD revealed his theories of "Jesus and the people from outer space," and the shrink went back to his mother and stepfather and said that David had a Christ complex and that he could have him committed if they wanted. The parents refused and sent McD off to London at his own request. After more troubles in London, on his return his parents said they would support him, but he had to dress in modern clothes and get a job and no more living in the past. A fight ensued, and he forced his grandmother to give him five dollars for the bus from New Jersey to Manhattan. There he moved in with his friend Jean Maria on East Third Street and set up a life as "Adele," his grandmother's name, a plain 1920s girl. Glenn O'Brien invited him to be on *TV Party,* his cable talk show of music and performance, on which Iggy Pop, Robert Mapplethorpe, David Byrne, David Bowie, and the B-52's would appear; it was there that Glenn also met a seventeen-year-old Jean-Michel Basquiat. At first, Jean-Michel was just in the audience; later, he manned the cameras and started typing in his own poems; and then he was on the show. McD told me he'd have to be uptown to film at midnight and they

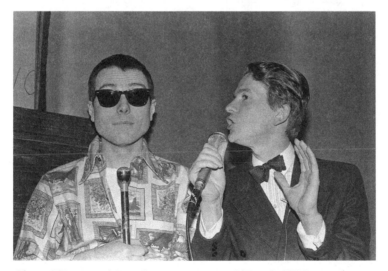

Glenn O'Brien and David McDermott on O'Brien's *TV Party,* a late-night cable show on which he interviewed well-known downtown figures, May 1, 1979

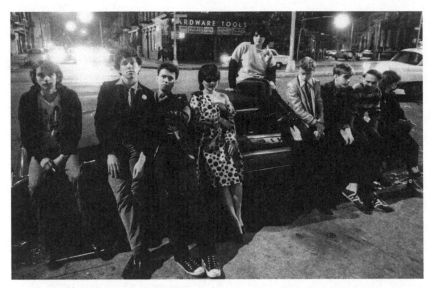

The punk crowd that took McDermott in, in front of CBGB's on the Bowery and Third: left to right, Harold, Kristian Hoffman, Diego Cortez, Anya Phillips, Lydia Lunch, James Chance, Jim Sclavunos, Bradley Field, and Liz Seidmann

only had a few hours for filming. "Of course, some of the people were on drugs there and had been up for twenty-four hours. I'd take a nap, bathe, and looked fresh."

The New York music-and-art scene of the East Village is where McD found acceptance. The rising gay-freedom culture of the 1970s thought him too weird. In the world of punk rock he found his place. When he told me this, I asked, "Do you like punk music?"

He grimaced. "Oh, it's horrible! But they're the only people who like me."

One morning after our ritual breakfast he asked, "What do you want to do with your life?"

"I want to be a famous artist," I earnestly replied.

"Oh, really!" His eyes widened. "That's perfect. I'm making an abstract painting for my mother's dining room. We can paint it together. But it has to be in orange because that's her favorite color." I later found out she commissioned the painting because she wanted some compensation for supporting him.

In his Bowery studio he pulled the Belgian linen on a large stretcher using carpet tacks. He placed a pot of water on an old Edison Electric hot plate from 1900 to boil rabbit-skin glue (which looked like sand) and proceeded to wet the linen with the pot of smelly liquid. As it dried, the linen became taut as a drum. After it dried, he opened a can of lead primer, stirring its denseness with a screwdriver. The can had a skull-and-crossbones on it with the word "Toxic" in red lettering.

In a week he called and said we were ready and I met him at his studio. He handed me a brush and had me start. On the dry, white, toxic coating I made a design on the colors he had prepared. My design was taken from a mid-century tiled lobby entrance I used to see back in my fashion-sketching days. I began by blocking out a circle, a triangle, and an amoeba shape. Then David laid colors in my lines and we went back and forth, working for a couple of weeks on the canvas. I was thrilled

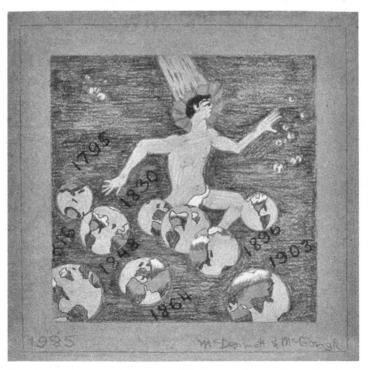

One of our drawings showing McD's theory of other Planet Earths in different time periods

to be working on what I thought of as a large painting. There was no formula to it, just our free expression. He would paint then I would add to it. He'd mix up a glaze, then put it into the shapes to change the colors slightly. When the painting was finally finished, we sat in the remaining sunlight and drank Welch's grape juice with packaged cookies. I found it easy to work with him, which added to his charm.

"Well," he said, pleased with our creation, "I guess this would be like an old Victorian artist who has been classically trained but who started making abstract paintings using all the old techniques but working in a modern way," he explained. "If I put an old date on it and it gets lost in the world, someone will think it's an antique and not throw it in the trash. You see, the old date saves it from obscurity." McD took glee in his statement and started to chuckle.

"Can't you see?" he excitedly expounded. (The sugar from the juice and cookies started kicking in.) "All time exists at the same time. There are parallel universes out there in other galaxies in different time periods. So, there are other Planet Earths out there. One is in 1928. Then another Planet Earth is in 1748! And another in 500 BC. And what I'm doing here by dating this painting—*our* painting—1947 is connecting with all these other planets in different portholes. Isn't that amazing?!" He went on for a while as I sipped the remaining grape juice and he ate the rest of the cookies. The afternoon was fading into dusk as the sun went down behind the Bowery Savings Bank. "Wait—I forgot to sign it!" He jumped out of his chair, picked up a brush, and in a passionate, childlike scrawl he wrote: "McDermott & McGough 1947."

He turned to look at me with an impish grin. "Now I have you forever."

6

McD continued to court me through the summer begging me to be his boyfriend. But after three months of waiting, he changed his tack. I was to meet him at the Mudd Club. When I arrived, I saw him and went up to greet him. He was standoffish and hardly spoke to me. He'd leave and go off to speak to someone else. When I followed him, he wouldn't introduce me or even look at me. I couldn't believe my friend was so rude after all the accolades he'd bestowed on me for months. He later told me his friend Margie, a statuesque blonde from Queens who dressed like a silent-movie star, with a jeweled headband and flowing dresses, gave him advice for the lovelorn. He told her of his unrequited love for me. She said, "Just ignore him. It always works for me." And indeed it worked for him: I required.

All children are taught to finger paint in school, enjoying the sensual feeling of the wet liquid between their fingers, laying that bright wetness on a large white piece of paper. Most children move on, away from the easel and paints. All but a few—they can't help but to keep going. I was one of those few; the pieces of paper became much more for me. I experienced a world I created, a safe haven in which I could live and dream, protected from my tormentors. When I met McDermott, his world was so well constructed—at least on paper—that it became immediately alluring, and I felt safe and cut off from a world I thought harsh and cruel.

"People like you, Peter, and they want to work with you," McDermott told me. "Nobody ever wanted to work with me. I tried to convince them, but I never succeeded. I never had the cushy jobs you had." Since the early 1970s he had made a living being a bank messenger, traveling on foot. They offered him a raise and a desk job, but he liked the freedom of working on foot, so he could drop by and visit friends in different neighborhoods.

We carried the finished painting for McDermott's mother on the train to New Jersey and walked it from the station through the kind of suburban neighborhoods I was so used to. Vivian had painted her front door bright orange enamel. To the door's right was a large, curved bay window where she had installed shelves to show off her collection of orange glazed pottery. Modernist Swedish-style furniture from Macy's

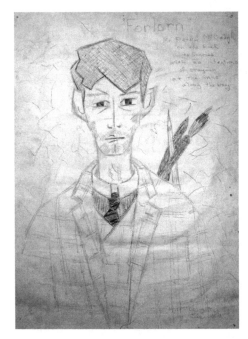

McDermott's 1980 drawing of me

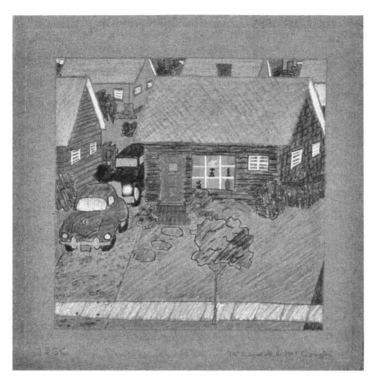

McDermott's mother's house in New Jersey with the orange door

was in the paneled living room where there were orange abstract paintings she had bought in Greenwich Village in the fifties, mixed with black African masks made out of plaster.

David pointed out the two similar abstract black-and-orange paintings in the living room. One was by an unknown artist. The other was painted by a fourteen-year-old David. Vivian had asked him to make a painting to go on the other wall. McD decided to make a version of one of the paintings she had bought in Greenwich Village, so he copied the style and palette and signed the other artist's name, Thomas, on it. "I wanted to make my mother look like she was an art collector."

McD then took me on a tour of the house showing me all the little extras that his mother had put in to make it look more modern. He said a girlfriend of hers went out with Billie Holiday's manager, so Vivian had gone with her to see the legendary jazz songbird, Lady Day. Vivian loved jazz and had all sorts of records, from Erroll Garner to Chet Baker. We sat around the painting as David and Vivian discussed its meaning. They turned to me but I had nothing to add. I felt embarrassed that I didn't have their vocabulary or their closeness. Vivian was a slim, petite replica of her son, with a soft, wavering voice. I found her to be elegant and intelligent, and I could see she wasn't exactly pleased that David had signed my name to the painting. But she was polite and took me in with a gentle smile. David begged her to let me see her wardrobe, so we went into her closet and she showed her many Chanel-style suits made from Vogue patterns, with nubby fabrics in soft gray or brown tones with silk trims that she wore into the city every day to work for Jack Dreyfus, the "Bond King."

"How's Walter?" she asked David as I looked over her wardrobe.

"Oh, he's all right. He moved to Florida."

"For good?" she questioned. David's family loved Walter.

"I don't know. We have to catch the bus."

We bade our adieus and I saw her slip him some money as she kissed his cheek.

"It was lovely to meet you, Peter." She held out her hand and looked intently at me. I didn't know what she was looking for, but she held my hand tightly for a few seconds as she gazed into my eyes.

On the bus back to Manhattan McD told me many stories about his interest in the past. "I saw old movies on TV and I thought, 'How come the present isn't as beautiful?' And how the world was going into a 'time death trap,' headed right into oblivion!" He continued, "I wasn't going to be cheated out of a great life. The modern world wants more and more and newer and newer. And they can't even deal with what they have!" His voice escalated, and I saw the disgruntled faces of the other passengers staring at us. He couldn't have cared less. "When my schoolteacher said to the class, 'You have to keep up or you'll be left behind,' well, I thought, as a young boy, I couldn't keep up with all of this—the modern world. So I made a conscious decision to go backwards." He stopped and looked at me intently, seeing if I was listening. "I looked for signs of the past everywhere, in places that were unchanged. When I was at Syracuse University I'd go to the library and look at the yearbooks from the twenties and study them. Then I found an old shop in an Italian neighborhood. In the back they had a record store that closed with the crash of '29. And still in the original sleeves they had records from 1928, 1929, and 1930. They had never been played so I was the first to hear those records on my crank Victrola. 'But,' I thought, 'these records weren't meant to be heard by the people of that time, they were actually meant for *me*!' They were telling me the secrets of time travel. I looked at this intact store for a porthole to the past. I even thought maybe they had a door in the back for me to go through time. Now, I wasn't time-traveling but I was certainly experimenting." And then he'd look at me intently followed by a mischievous giggle. I had never been privy to such insane and, in some ways, inspiring discourse. As the bus pulled into Port Authority, he recounted a story of how when he was ten years old, he had seen an ad in the real-estate section of the local papers: "For Sale: 1928 pink marble mansion. Built for one million dollars. Yours for ten thousand dollars."

"Look at this!" he had excitedly showed his mother. "We can sell our tiny house and live in a mansion! It's only ten thousand dollars!"

"We don't have the furniture to fill such a big house, David," his mother explained.

"We don't have to get it all at once!" he replied.

"It's much too expensive to heat."

"We don't have to heat it in the summer. And it has so many fireplaces!"

Then she firmly let him know they weren't moving and there would be no further discussion. "After that," he leaned in and whispered to me, "I knew they weren't to be trusted."

After a few months, Walter had changed jobs and come back from Florida by way of Texas and we all moved into the Arlington Hotel on Fifth Avenue and Twenty-Fifth Street off Madison Square. This hotel was now a sort of SRO for transients. You could see how opulent it had once been by the putti hanging off the ceiling cornices in the dining room, a space now used for storing the hotel's mattresses. Our room had an old fireplace and looked out on a brick wall, but was surprisingly intact, even the bath.

Neither David nor Walter had any money or a job, so I supported both of them. That is, until the police raided Danceteria and shut it down. All the employees were arrested and handcuffed to one another, and we spent the night in a large jail cell downtown along with street thugs and junkies. When they let us out in the morning, David was there waiting.

Through working the night shift at Danceteria, I came across many children of the night. One person hovering around my ticket booth was Johnny Rudo, aka Johnny Rudowitz. A cute button of a person with barbershop-cut raven hair and large black eyes, he couldn't buy me drinks, so he paid me compliments. Johnny lived just below Bryant Park. Most parks after dark in Manhattan were for sex cruising or drugs—or both. He invited me to his two-story loft for drinks. I don't think he was so pleased when I showed up with David and Walter. It was a vast, gutted floor of an old townhouse with no walls except for a kitchen and a bath, and a small wooden staircase leading to another floor. Upstairs was an intact Victorian apartment, complete with a telephone box on the wall and original nineteenth-century wallpaper. I saw McDermott's eyes widen as he took in the place and its possibilities.

He turned to Johnny. "You live here all by yourself?" Already I could hear the wheels in motion, as I could no longer afford the rent at the Arlington.

"No," said Johnny, "I have a roommate. He's an artist, Kenny Scharf, and his friend Keith Haring is here all the time." He looked over at me. "I'd rather have you as my roommate." McDermott looked at me, smiling. "Oh, no," I thought.

David walked over to me as Walter claimed Johnny's attention.

"Listen—you have to seduce Johnny."

"What?" I whispered. "Forget it!"

"Don't get upset. You have to. We need this place to live. And he really likes you. We've been in that expensive dump of a hotel and we are out of money." I was thinking: "You mean *I* ran out of money."

"Take him up to the top of the Empire State Building and just be friendly."

Well, I did just that and we kissed in the moonlight. What was I going to do with another boyfriend? I spent the night on the sofa bed with Johnny in the loft since he gave Kenny the upstairs, but it was uneventful. The next day David and Walter arrived with their suitcases. Kenny was away, and Johnny nervously paced the room for Kenny's arrival.

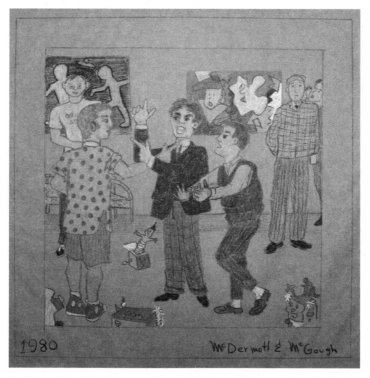

At Johnny Rudo's, left to right: Keith Haring, Kenny Scharf, David McDermott, Johnny Rudo, me, and Walter, during the fight for the loft

"Don't worry, Johnny, I'll take care of him," said McD.

David went on a cleaning spree and mopped and vacuumed the downstairs when Johnny was out. He went through a pile of clothes that were strewn all over the floor and separated the wool and cotton from the polyester and double knits. A pair of 1970s peace-symbol polyester pants from Sears made it into the bad pile. He bundled it all up in a Vera designer sheet and took it across the street next to a garbage can. When Johnny returned, he was pleased to see the loft so clean.

"Wait—where are all my clothes?"

"Here they are!" David proudly showed how he had ironed and folded his clothes and neatly put them away.

"Where's the rest?"

"Well," chirped David, "I only kept the good ones. I mean, those other ones weren't even good enough to use as rags!"

While a heated argument ensued and escalated, I looked out the window across the street to see a crowd going through the polyester pile. A day later Kenny showed up with Keith Haring. They were friendly at first, but the friendliness turned sour when Kenny saw that David had washed the graffiti off the refrigerator and removed the glued plastic figures.

"What the fuck is going on here?" Kenny screamed. "What are you doing here?"

Then McD started screaming that Johnny wanted both of them out because they were so mean to him. Then it really started to explode, and a fight began. I looked over at Johnny who was sitting on the sofa biting his nails. As far as I can remember, Kenny went upstairs or departed.

Soon Walter and Johnny started sleeping together. That night I heard Walter whisper to David, lying on the other sofa, "You and Peter have to leave."

"But why? I worked so hard cleaning this mess of all its garbage. It's not fair!"

"Kenny pays most of the rent," Walter whispered back to McD. "I'll stay here with John and you and Peter can go to Wardle House upstate for two weeks while I look for another place, and then you can return."

Those two weeks would become almost a year.

Kenny recently told me that he had to leave the property after he had a large booze-and-drug-filled party to which some man who had been stabbed in the park came climbing up the stairs bleeding and then slumped down into a corner. The partygoers thought it was performance art. Later someone saw that he was really bleeding and called the police.

7

David's country house was a two-floor, twenty-five-room apartment he rented for twenty-five dollars a month above the Wardle Drug Store on Warren Street in Hudson. In exchange for the low rent David had agreed to bring part of the apartment up to code with heating, electricity, and plumbing. I saw no sign of that agreement. The apartment had no kitchen but every possible 1910 luxury in the bathrooms, though nothing worked. The only source of water (other than the glass bottles of sulfured Saratoga Spring water still there after seventy years—yes, we drank it all) was a cold-water drip from a pantry sink faucet.

"See," David would say, holding up a full white-enamel bucket. "Now that took just about an hour to fill, and we can empty this and fill it up again." I'm surprised that I didn't just bolt for the train back to New York. But Walter had said it was only for two weeks. And I wanted an interesting life, and McD was more interesting than anyone else I knew. The water was used for bathing in a washbasin by the only source of heat, the fireplace in the living room. As the winter came upon us, the only place to cook, read, sleep, and eat was the living room, and the 1940s sofa turned into a bed. We tried sleeping in a bedroom upstairs, but I realized it was too cold when I reached for my

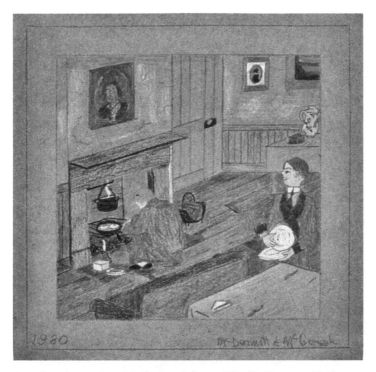

David is setting the table for breakfast at Wardle House in Hudson
while I cook eggs in the fireplace.

bedside glass of water only to find it had frozen into a glass of ice. David
had many projects going on at the same time around the house. There
were big plans to remove an old floral painted glass ceiling from the
flower market back in New York and install it in the ceiling he ripped
out in the apartment the year before. That never happened. I tended to
the house and learned to cook our meals—over the floorboards McD
ripped up—in the only working fireplace. McD had a habit of ripping
out the top layer of the newer flooring covering older, wider floorboards underneath. Walter and David had moved the furniture from
the Avenue B apartment into the two floors of the house. One room
he called his "Manhattan apartment" which consisted of modern and
"art decorative" furniture. He gave me a lecture when I called it deco.
"That's not even a word! It was completely made up in the seventies.
It's either 'art decoratif,' 'art modern,' or 'streamline.' Never use the

word 'deco'! That's tacky. And it's 'drapery,' not 'drapes'! That's as bad as saying 'dem,' 'dese,' and 'dose.' I read it in Emily Post."

Once I realized we were there for a while, I set up a corner of the warm room to paint in. I'd make preliminary drawings, and if they weren't up to my self-inflicted standards I'd bunch them into a ball. McD found them and asked why I destroyed such beautiful drawings. "They're not good enough," I'd sigh. "Well, you can't do that! I can't draw like this," he'd lament. "Every work you do belongs to me, too, since we're now partners. So, no more destroying your work." And that was the start of building my confidence.

We never fought about the art. He seemed to like everything I painted, and I certainly liked his style. In New York he used to do a few portraits of gays in the Lower East Side art world. I watched him do one on Halloween. He asked the sitter to buy a paint kit and canvas.

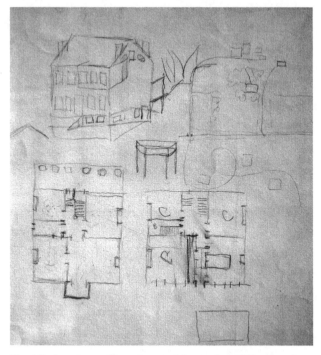

David's drawings of how he would transform Wardle
House into a palace, with more staircases and other details

David laid the canvas on the floor of the man's apartment and went to work. When he finished—to the awe of the sitter—he collected his two-hundred-dollar fee, which was a fortune for us, and we immediately went to eat. He would also show me his elaborate drawings of floor plans of Wardle House, detailing how he was going to make it over into a showplace. That would lead to a two-hour monologue of his theories on the history of decoration.

We'd often roam around Hudson. In the afternoon we'd take the back alleyways while David gave one of his many monologues on architecture, pointing out doors and cornices. We had learned to walk the backstreets because on the main street we were ducking rocks thrown at us from mocking children.

On one of our walks a comical elderly figure came up to us and complimented us on our dress. She invited us to a church service the next morning. "Ten bells, lambs," she said, expecting us to go. We later went on our own to the Seventh-day Adventist church dinners because they were vegans, we were hungry, and the food was free. We had two pairs of Brooks Brothers shoes that David's mother bought him, and two 1930s suits from the boys' section we'd switch daily to pretend we had a wardrobe. Our figures, made especially boyish from skipped meals, fit easily into the junior wear, if you ignored my wrists and ankles sticking out. We had some shirts with highly starched detachable collars that made the shine and the wrinkles from the rayon suits less noticeable. We were constantly sewing buttons and patching little holes to keep them going. We were meticulous in our "penny millionaire" style.

We felt we were making a statement by our very existence. Some elders would come up to us asking if we were in the military because we had barbershop haircuts cropped closely around the sides and back. We wore old belted coats and homburg hats. When we wore black frock coats and dark hats on the Lower East Side of Manhattan, the Hasidim would drive by in yellow school buses, stop, open the door, and yell, "We're going over the Williamsburg Bridge—do you want a ride?" Or kids in the neighborhood would yell out "Fucking kikes!" or "Faggots!" Some thought us Amish. Others thought we were older than we were because of our dress. We were anarchists of the past. McDermott relished the attention. I didn't. I didn't like the constant interruptions from strangers: "Are you in a movie?" "Why are you dressed like that?"

Hudson in 1980 was a quiet town with a couple of restaurants that offered a five-dollar dinner we could not afford. Along the main street there were many outmoded shops—a pen shop, a ladies' department store, and one antiques shop, Bobbie's Antiques, next to many empty stores that moved to the mall on a highway. McD was working on transferring his unemployment from his singing and being the master of ceremonies at a nightclub in Queens—which I never saw—to the Hudson office. For his interview in the local office he wore morning clothes and a top hat. "Are you getting married?" someone asked him at the door.

I tagged along, hoping they would give him some money. The middle-aged man who handled the transfer was decked out in a wide-lapelled green-pastel three-piece suit. Going over McD's application, he looked up and asked, "So you're in show business?"

"Yes," David answered seriously.

"Yes," the man mimicked. "Hmm . . ." He hummed as he went over the paperwork. "I don't think there is much work for you in this field in Hudson."

David shrugged. The man cleared his throat. "Well . . . I've been told I should go into show business."

"Really!" spouted David.

"Yes. I've been told I have a good radio voice," the man continued. " 'Why wait till winter to get those new tires?' " His voice fell a few octaves while he did his mock commercial.

And they went on forever, chatting and chuckling about making it in showbiz like two pieces of ham yammering. I was ready to hit them both with the stapler on the man's desk. After a while that seemed eternal, he looked us both over through his wire aviator frames, stamped the card, and handed it to David. "Maybe something will open up in Albany. I'll see you in a few weeks." We finally had our meal ticket.

The next few months in Hudson were idyllic, and winter became spring, so we could move about and sleep in another room. We'd make our breakfast on the fire in the morning, read or paint a little, and then roam the back alleys, picking bouquets of flowering weeds and, as usual, seeing what trash we could drag back to the house. I loved these walks down the rather romantic backstreets, with small run-down houses shaded by crooked trees and guarded by rusted cast-iron fences above old rosebushes, frozen in time.

We'd peer into the windows of our favorite empty house (which strangely always had a mowed lawn), through the torn lace curtains and the faded green shade with its rotted silk tassel, misshapen by time and pulled by gravity. Beyond the menagerie of the window coverings we spied a rose-pattern-papered dining room. We'd each look through a window, calling out to one another to notice the elaborately painted radiator in different colors in the corner, the matching 1900s dining-room set from a mail-order catalogue, the empty glass fruit bowl on the sideboard below a print of flowers in a gold frame, hanging by a silk cord from a decorative picture rail.

On one of our daily walks looking for free antiques in the back-alley garbage piles, we ventured into an antiques store just to peruse what they had. While I looked over the antiques, David started talking to two women who were quietly whispering, having tea in the back of the shop. One of the women in particular seemed a little odd to me, somewhat resembling Prince Charles in drag. She was wearing a proper "English lady"–styled outfit of a pleated wool plaid skirt below the knee, sensible low-heeled shoes, opaque hose, and a cashmere twin set with a string of pearls—all topped off with a cream puff of light auburn hair.

David called me over, introducing me, "This is my partner, Peter."

The lady in question raised her hand to mine as she balanced the teacup in another. "Hello," she greeted me in the softest voice, "how do you do? I'm Dawn. Dawn Langley Simmons," as her hand engulfed mine.

Shaking her limp, soft, and quite large, ringed hand, I replied, "How do you do?" in my best Noël Coward manner. As Dawn sipped her tea from the delicate flowered cup, I noticed her gaudy cocktail ring which sparkled in the afternoon light. I had never talked to a trans person before, other than a few words with Marsha P. Johnson, a black trans woman on Christopher Street. Marsha was at the Stonewall riot of 1969.

Dawn seemed quite "high-tone" compared with the others I had met in the West Village. She put on quite a refined pitch, almost a whisper. "We're neighbors, I hear?" she softly asked me, smiling. I later learned that Dawn was the love-child son of Vita Sackville-West's chauffeur. The English actress Margaret Rutherford, famous for her Miss Marple performances, had befriended Dawn, who thought of her as a second mother. In 1980, Dawn was no ordinary person for Hudson, or anywhere else. She was a published author and had written a memoir about being a hermaphrodite and giving birth to a beautiful black baby girl, who at the time was a teenager attending the local Catholic school. Her story was later questioned. The hearsay and gossip were that her late African-American husband went mad and ran down the main street naked, ending up in a mental hospital.

Dawn lived right around the corner from us in an 1810 Federal brick house filled with beautiful, although not-in-the-best-condition, antiques. She said her friend Isabel Whitney gave some to her. We only visited her once—and once was enough.

Dawn greeted us at the door, and the overpowering odor of ammoniated cat piss slapped me in the face as I entered. There were cats everywhere! I spotted three on the mantel next to two enormous cracked French paste vases. There were six more cats on the sofa, with a few peeking out from under it. Ten or more were on the floor, fighting or lounging and scratching the sagging Empire divan. I could hear more cats fighting on the stairs. Four or five of them came up to me meowing, leaving heaps of fur on my trouser legs.

"Oh, I do have a few cats, don't I?" Dawn shyly suggested.

When Dawn's back was to me, I'd shoo them away, and pushed one that was clawing up my pants leg. There were also overflowing litter boxes and cat poo lying about. It was beyond soap and water. We didn't stay long. "My God, couldn't she open a window?" I asked David as we gasped for fresh air outside. I never knew what became of Dawn. But I can still smell her pretty house.

Since we had no electricity, and therefore no television, I started going to the library and reading as much as I could. The library, a former eighteenth-century mental hospital, was a regular stop for us. I started with Henry James, then E. M. Forster and W. Somerset Maugham; I went through the Time-Life series on artists like Duchamp, Cézanne, and van Gogh. We also rented reels of silent films and played them on the projector in the church's basement following meetings of the Bible study group. The group wasn't so thrilled with McD's idea that the twelve apostles were Jesus's boyfriends. "It's just a theory!" David would exclaim to defend himself. Two transplanted beret-wearing Greenwich Village beatniks, George and Janie Davis, would share their sandwiches with us. Seeing how we devoured them, they started bringing us each one of our own. David always attended church wherever he lived. "It's social, Peter," he'd explain as I grumbled at the idea of going. "It's how one meets people."

He preferred a Protestant service rather than "those cursing Catholics." And he called Episcopalians "high Catholics," and not because the local church organist was a pot dealer. McD gave out the Wardle drug store's number as his own, and they politely left us messages.

One day there was a message from the Wardle drug store from his old friend Glenn O'Brien. Glenn was producing a film with the twenty-year-old Jean-Michel Basquiat. We went down to the train station to call Glenn collect from a pay phone. He asked David to come to the city to play himself. They would arrange for two train tickets and give him two hundred dollars as a fee. We went down to the station to collect the tickets the next morning. The man at the ticket window said there were no tickets sent. McD was livid and criticized the train company for being so unprofessional. "I'm starring in a movie and you're ruining my chances!" he screamed to a blank-faced attendant.

When the train arrived, he grabbed our suitcase and pushed me onto the train. "Get on! Get on!" he screeched.

Out of my window I saw the stationmaster go up to the conductor to tell him of our boarding. I had never seen such rebellion before. We had no credit cards or any money on us that would pay for the fare. As the train started to leave the station, the conductor came to our seats, bluntly asking us for our tickets. David went on about how incompetent the trains were, and they had lost our tickets. That only annoyed the man more. He barked at us to get off at the next station. As I stood up, David harshly whispered, "Sit down—we're not leaving!"

"I don't want to get arrested."

"Why do you always have to be so dramatic, Peter?"

I was about to continue arguing when I heard the conductor yelling, "What are you two still doing here? You can't ride the train for free!" Other passengers put down their books to stare at the commotion.

"We're not going anywhere!" McD screeched back. "It's the train company's fault! Our tickets are lost, and we have to get to New York today. I'm in a movie!"

"I don't care if you're landing on the moon—you'll get off at the next stop."

My nervousness grew as I sat silent. We came to a stop near a dirt road that crossed the tracks, and the train waited. It stood so long people were getting annoyed, and there was no conductor to complain to. Then from the window I saw two police cars with blinking lights pulled up on either side of the train.

"Oh . . . no!" I cried out.

"Leave this to me, Peter," David said as I buried my face in my hands.

Then two sheriffs boarded the train. One, with a big belly, looked like Jackie Gleason in a cop movie. "What do you boys think you're doing?" he said, leaning his face into ours.

David went on to explain that we were waiting for our tickets and that the train company failed us.

"Well, where you boys headed?" he asked us.

"The island of Manhattan," David said.

" 'The island of Manhattan,' " the cop slowly repeated, mockingly.

The whole train car was now standing to get a look at the scenario playing out.

"Now get your bags and get off this train!" the sheriff's voice boomed. "You have a long walk back to the island of Manhattan."

We immediately jumped up, took our suitcase from above, and departed.

The train left, and the sheriff looked at us from his car window, jerked his thumb and said, "Now beat it!," and drove off.

We walked in silence along the tracks till we arrived at the next train station. We went into the old station in Poughkeepsie and David went to the counter to explain. The elderly man listened and wrote a note that read, "These two boys are visiting their mother and their tickets didn't come. She has the tickets, is waiting at Grand Central, and will hand them to the conductor."

"Just show this to the conductor and it'll be fine," he said warmly.

McD called Glenn and told him when we'd be arriving and to have someone meet us with tickets. We must have looked like old theater people in our getups. We sat on the train and showed the note to a confused conductor. He shrugged and gave us seats. In Grand Central, Glenn's assistant was waiting for us.

"Do you have the tickets?" McD asked.

"No—come on, let's go."

I swallowed my rage but was relieved someone had met us and followed him downtown in a taxi to the set. The director, photographer Edo Bertoglio, and his wife, the stylist and designer Maripol, were across the street on Astor Place with Glenn and a camera set up, waiting for McD's scene with Jean-Michel. They threw him right into it.

McD was dressed up with a homburg and a high starched collar. His lines were about how horrible the modern world is. "David—here are your lines, but say what you want," directed Glenn, who knew David so well that the lines he wrote were exactly as McD spoke. The punk actor who was supposed to do the scene with Basquiat and McD wasn't there. McD said he would run to Klaus Nomi's apartment to ask him to fill in. He came back empty-handed. "I knocked on his door and he said, 'Go away—I'm not well.' " Klaus died three years later, in 1983, of AIDS. He was thirty-nine, and one of the first we knew to die of it.

There was a girl with green hair whom I knew from Danceteria walking by just then. We grabbed her and did the scene. She was happy to get the fifty-dollar fee. They later named the film *Downtown 81* and finally released it in 2001.

We did not stay long afterwards, since we were sleeping feet to feet on Chuck's couch in his studio apartment on West Eighth Street, until it became too much for the small room to hold us and we headed once again for Hudson.

Back home in Hudson, we were running out of the wood flooring McD tore up to burn for our fire, but David found a large dead tree in the alleyway someone had cut down. He convinced me to help him drag the tree full of branches home, just a few blocks away, but the weight of the tree meant it took an hour to drag it through the alley, and it scratched all the parked cars along the way. We finally pulled it into the ground floor of the house, and David started to saw it into pieces. Most of the tree was out the open door onto the sidewalk for a few days. The tree had the street talking, and days later we were evicted with a notice to depart the now condemned property. No heating, electricity, or plumbing, said the served papers.

We saw that the top floor of a house across the street was for rent. It was named the Curtiss House after its first owners. For three hundred a month we rented the six large rooms on the top floor. Of course, we never paid the rent. McD opened the barn behind it by breaking the lock and emptied out the mounds of furniture and set up the house. A woman in the office below handled the rent for the owner of a modeling agency. She called him and said we hadn't been paying and had taken the furniture out of the barn. He asked if we were destroying the property. When the woman relayed that we were restoring the brick path that went around the house and that we regularly cut the lawn, he told her to just leave us be.

Huge pizza ovens dominated the barn. McD was trying to move them when a truck went by and asked what we were doing with them. David offered them the pizza ovens and they took them. There was also a lot of scrap metal there, and we went to visit a scrap man on the north side of town. He came over and paid us for the metal. So now we had a little money.

About a week later some tough-looking Italian guys who looked right out of a Little Italy social club drove up and started screaming for their pizza ovens. I turned and yelled up to the house for David to come down. When he did, their fury had peaked. McD told them a man drove up and took the ovens, saying they were his. When asked about the metal, he said it had gone to a scrap man. "What are these guys, the daisy-chain gang?" one grunted. They forced us into their car and off we went to the scrap yard. When we arrived, they went up to the man who'd bought the metal and demanded the return of it and the pizza ovens. The man said he didn't ever have the ovens. The guys were screaming about a thick sheet of metal about the size of a large rug. They wanted it. I looked at the man and he lowered his eyes as a secret gesture. I looked down and saw we were all standing on the large sheet of metal. After about twenty minutes they left in a huff knowing that they had lost the property. As we walked back home, I saw smoke coming from the lower part of the barn. I went around to the street and saw a broken window with more smoke coming out.

"David!" I screamed. "The barn is on fire!"

He came running and saw the smoke. He then ran down the block in the middle of Warren Street, screaming, "Fire! Fire!" until he got to the fire station. Soon two fire trucks came roaring up to the house. This excitement brought all the neighborhood kids to the yard looking for some fun. The firemen put out the small fire and said it was arson: someone had dropped a burning rag in the window. After they left, our yard was full of kids from neighborhoods far and wide. McD ordered them to get out so he could close the back gate, but the kids weren't having it. They were mad that he wouldn't let them pick pears from a tree in the yard. "They're not ripe yet!" he'd scream. "Get them in a few weeks." But they wouldn't leave so he turned on the garden hose and started to spray them. But since it was summer, they loved it even more and started pushing each other to get in the spray from the hose. Finally, they left. We found out years later that by giving away the ovens, we had stopped these crooks conning unsuspecting people who might have wanted to open a pizza joint.

The church beatniks gave us packages of zucchini, collard greens, and peas and we planted a garden after tilling the yard with the manure from the barn. We ended up with a crop of collard greens that grew knee-high. David's grandmother said not to pick them till after the first frost. We gave away many large collards to the members of the Shiloh Baptist Church next door. We also left a few baskets of pears after we attended a service there.

A few weeks before Christmas in 1980 we took a bus from Hudson to Albany because David wanted to visit his friend Justin Hoag. One summer, two years before, while walking up Warren Street in his usual attire of white linen and a boater hat, David passed a similarly dressed younger man. As they walked by each other they both tipped their straw hats. David abruptly turned into the alleyway to run around back to the main street and introduce himself. As the young man did the same, they ended up introducing themselves in the alleyway. Justin Hoag was living in a large apartment on Warren Street, and he invited David there for tea.

"My first impression was that I couldn't believe the grandeur of his place with all these antiques," David told me. "After a while I noticed the furniture was mostly broken including the sofa which was missing a leg and was propped up by bricks. And there were beer bottles and empty pizza boxes strewn all over the place."

We made our way to downtown Albany and found Justin's address. He was living in an old efficiency apartment with a bed that rolled out

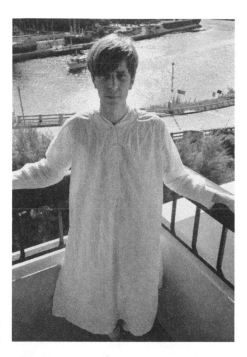

Our friend Justin Hoag on
a balcony in his nightshirt
in the late eighties

from under a bookshelf. We found him lounging there in a mad disarray of plates of leftover food, books, clothes, and some marijuana para-
phernalia. He was wearing striped pajamas and a fifties speckled sports
jacket and drinking from a cracked yellowed beer stein. I surmised it
was vodka from the empty bottle on his littered bed. In his other hand
was the longest cigarette I'd ever seen, from which he exhaled a billow
of smoke. A pack of Benson & Hedges 100's in gold packaging lay on
the rumpled sheets. He was reed thin, with messy, badly bleached blond
hair, and an elegant acne-scarred face. It looked like he had been in that
bed for a long while. He put out his cigarette gently, trying not to topple
the tower of nicotine butts resting on a marble ashtray among the ruins.
He was like a satyr—all sex and bacchanalia—under a cloud of smoke.

A *New York Post* was on the table with the headline that John Lennon had just been shot and killed outside the Dakota apartments. "Yes,
terrible news," Justin said. "But if it had been Garbo, then I really
would have to go into mourning."

I sat there as David and he rambled on about mutual friends and living in Hudson. I took in my surroundings, the chipped and cracked glamour. I was impressed by how he had put all these discarded and worn antiques together so well, creating a Miss Havisham look. I had heard so much about this person, his eviction from Hudson and all the problems he had caused. I let the two of them speak without trying to join in, since I had only been living with McDermott for a few months.

When Justin found out we weren't in Wardle House anymore but living across the street at the Curtiss House, he went on excitedly about what a magnificent edifice it was. "I've always dreamed of living there, coming down the staircase in a Greek Revival tea gown, or morning dress. The front door has been left open overnight, and the dead leaves would be scattered about the hallway; then a great wind would come up and the leaves would engulf me." He burst out in a cackle.

On a weekend visit to Hudson in the seventies, David and Walter had discovered Justin had broken into Wardle House and moved in with all his belongings. He had a small television wired through the house and connected by many electrical cords to an outlet in the basement of the drug store below in order to watch reruns of *I Love Lucy*. After the initial shock David wasn't so annoyed, because finally his twenty-five rooms were furnished.

Justin had two looks for two ways of making money. One look was the "tattered Victorian" with a smashed-in top hat, a moth-eaten morning suit, yellowed stiff shirt and detachable collar ("Original starch," he'd quip), broken dancing pumps with frayed bows, and dirty white kid gloves. "Who cares if it's broken or dirty? At least it's original!" was Justin's motto. He'd mill around town, usually at the flea market or antiques shops, in this getup, with his usual paper shopping bag on his arm ("This is a good one—vintage Bonwit Teller—feel the heaviness of the paper!"), plus the eternal lit cigarette hanging between his bony, stained fingers and a blue paper coffee cup. I rarely saw him without one of these items, or all three. He used all sorts of lingo such as "schmancy," a mixture of "shiny" and "fancy"; "witchy," referring to something good; and "dreck," bad merchandise, or "merch."

Justin's other look was quite the opposite. It was his idealization of a 1970s porn actor. First of all, his hair was bleached the color of a canary, with bangs that his blue eyes would peer out from under and cut with a mullet, giving him the look of Florence Henderson on *The Brady Bunch,* one of his favorite TV shows. He said his mullet was a nod to the eighteenth century. He had wide shoulders and slim hips, which he'd accentuate by wearing bold-colored 1970s running shorts with contrasting piping; added to that were knee-length tube socks, vintage sneakers, and a cut-off mesh football jersey to show off his slim waistline. The Victorian shabby-genteel look was for a daytime of buying and selling antiques. The other look was his night and weekend look. "I'm a lady of the evening and I'm at your mercy," he'd snort, with a laugh. If he didn't have enough money from selling antiques, he'd go up to Fifty-Third Street and Third Avenue to hustler bars with such names as Cowboys & Cowgirls and Rounds to make the rent. It was always packed with young men at the beginning and end of a month. This corner was so famous that the Ramones sang about it in their song "53rd & 3rd." Justin would go back and forth constantly between Manhattan and upstate. When he didn't have a penny, he'd hitchhike. If he needed funds, he'd go up to the top of Main Street in Catskill in his porn look and stand in front of a tattoo parlor to turn tricks.

Justin showed up in Hudson one day when we were living in the Curtiss House. He came through the front door and ran up the stairs. I was just making dinner and we invited him to stay. David served our vegetarian meal on Victorian plates. Justin took one look at the dish and said loudly, "This needs to be reheated and served on a plate that is not cracked! Look at this dreck you served me," and he pushed the plate away from him. In an instant, McD blew up and screamed, "Then get the hell out of here!" as he took the plate of food and threw it out the front window, where it crashed next to a cannon on the front lawn. Justin just stared at him, saying, "Temper, temper," and left. Another time, when McD and I were out, he opened the front door (we never locked it) and took what he said was his "merch." Justin would also get odd jobs decorating rich lady friends' apartments, but when he found himself low on cash he'd sneak over while they were gone, move the furniture, and roll up the Persian carpets to resell them to dealers. He once bought a gold-framed Hudson River School painting by Sanford Gifford for ten dollars in Albany, sold it, and then stole it back later to sell again. His sticky fingers were found all over his "merch."

I had set up a very small studio in Curtiss House in a room on the second floor with bay windows where I would work late mornings for the light. One day I looked down and saw David speaking to the neighbors next door on their back porch. He came up and said they had invited us over. When we arrived, I thought they looked ancient. I was twenty-three and they were probably fortyish. The dominant personality was Edward Avedisian. He was a barrel-chested Armenian from Boston who was heralded in the sixties as one of the up-and-coming

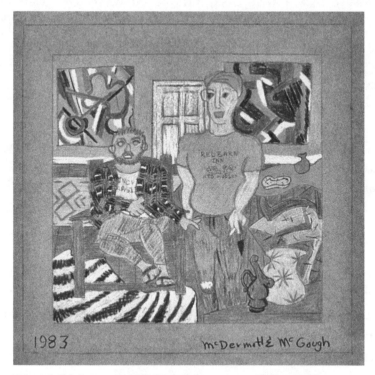

Edward Avedisian seated, left, with his partner, Judson Baldwin, standing, in their house in Hudson, with Edward's paintings on wall

artists, along with Warhol. Edward boasted he had shown Warhol how to mix up his fluorescent colors. He also traded paintings with Andy. After much coercing he finally told me it was a double Silver Elvis that he traded with Warhol and then later traded for another artist's watercolors. He became livid when I chuckled at his art trade. In the beginning of Edward's career, he said, Henry Geldzahler, then a curator at the Metropolitan Museum, was his confidant; but he later was dropped for David Hockney. Geldzahler's old boyfriend Christopher Scott, who's standing in the famous Hockney portrait of the two of them, lived down the street from Edward in a house that was under construction for years.

We sat in Avedisian's kitchen with its golden oak table and chairs from a 1900 Sears, Roebuck catalogue. Bright Fiestaware plates and Roseville pottery lay about. They had painted the refrigerator purple. "He's like the Norma Desmond of the art world," David whispered.

In the middle of the table, in an old ironstone platter, was the largest mound of marijuana I had ever seen. We shared a big joint with them until McD stood up and mumbled an incoherent apology about Jesus and the people from outer space and walked backwards out of their house. They never offered us a joint again. I would visit them later in the week and the mound was almost gone. They lived off pennies while Edward sold a painting here and there. We had only three paintings we were working on. Edward had no qualms about hating our work, and I think he disliked us, but he was desperate for company. We were his only connection to the New York art world. And being gay helped. He once barked at us, "You're not real artists—if someone brought a roll of wallpaper you'd drop everything to look at it!" Unflinching, David replied, "Well, it would depend on how good the wallpaper was." Edward mostly grumbled about the art world and how after he died he'd be famous. That didn't happen. He'd rail about a young artist named Julian Schnabel—"some kid Castelli's showing. He thinks he's so great because he put antlers in his paintings." I had no idea who he was talking about. Avedisian had lost it all—a townhouse, paintings, etc.—in a divorce after he met his partner, Judson, cruising the piers on the West Side Highway. Judson was a big blond southerner constantly smoking unfiltered Camels who liked to show me nude pictures of himself in his prime. Edward had a son in Manhattan who looked like a beautiful, pale youth from an eighteenth-century painting.

Our idyllic, small-town country life ended abruptly when a friend of Avedisian's, composer Aaron Copland's private chef, bought the Greek Revival manor and we had to depart. They wanted us to pay rent. The previous owner offered us the house for thirty thousand dollars. We didn't have thirty dollars, much less thirty thousand. We emptied the house of anything that wasn't bolted down. "We won't leave them a crumb," McD angrily stated. Years later, we heard from Avedisian that the new owner and his boyfriend had both died of AIDS.

8

It was July 1981, we had no place to live, and so we returned to New York. Arriving in Penn Station, David called a high-school friend, Roseanne, who let us stay on her sofa for a month. I soon learned the unspoken etiquette that when one stays in a friend's house, whether on the sofa or in a room, one washes the dishes from the night before (dishwashing machines were rare downtown), departs early before the host wakes up, and returns after dinner.

David called his mother, Vivian, who offered to help us get an apartment. That weekend, we took the bus to New Jersey to have Sunday dinner at her house. His grandmother Nana was there, and after dinner she and Vivian sat to have a talk with David. I sat with his stepfather, Bill, as I watched them out of the corner of my eye. "You need to get serious and make some money, David," Vivian advised.

"I'm an artist and we're just starting out."

"I know, honey," Nana interrupted. "I know you're a talented genius. But we can't go on supportin' you. We're not rich people. And I'm livin' on a budget."

"Daddy and I can help you and Peter to get settled with this place, but you have to get to work." I could see David's face starting to twitch.

Suddenly he burst out, livid, "You know, I just came here with Peter for a nice dinner, and you two turned it into an attack!"

"No one is attacking you," his mother said.

"Yeah," Nana chimed in, "Mother and I work very hard for our money, and we can't continue . . ."

David stood up and cried out, "Just give me the check and I'll go!"

Vivian gave him the check as Nana continued, "You're so ungrateful, that's what it is." Then, swiftly changing her tune: "Now, honey, be reasonable."

"We're leaving! Come on, Peter."

I stood up, thanked his family, and said my goodbyes, thinking how this was right out of some southern gothic tale by Tennessee Williams. We walked silently through the suburban streets and waited on the highway for a bus to Manhattan. David told me another story about how Nana had a brass figure of a hooded monk and when you turned it around it became a penis. When David told her it was a dildo, she screamed, "It belonged to Ray's brother—he was a sailor!" Ray was Nana's third husband. Nana was certainly an interesting character. She'd spout, "I've got my own kind of religion." I could tell because on her coffee table were an assortment of old pamphlets. One was called "The Flag Speaks," another was about space aliens. McD seemed to be a mix of his intellectual, atheist mother and his religious "free thinker" grandmother.

Walter was back in our lives, staying with us at Bradley and Kristian's on the Bowery again. Walter and I went to the Mudd Club one night and snorted heroin with an old Warhol superstar. We stayed out late, and it was near dawn when we wandered back to the corner room where David was asleep. It seemed that as soon as I put my head on the pillow, David was up.

"Come on, Walter, get up! Wake up, Peter, we're moving into our new place on Avenue A today!"

"NO! Let us sleep more," we begged. With the noise David was making getting ready, we soon dragged ourselves up.

While McD was down the hall Walter offered me some cocaine he had in his pocket. "This'll help," he added. I was just about to lean down and snort it when the door opened and McD walked in.

"What are you doing? *Drugs!*" he screamed as his eyes popped. "Walter! What are you doing?" Now the veins in his forehead were bulging. He continued screaming: "Peter, if you're going to be with me and we're going to build a life together, there are going to be *no* drugs! I'm not interested in drugs. Only tacky people do drugs! Drugs are for sick people!" I certainly felt sick. "So, you better make up your mind right now—a life with me or a life with drugs!" Still feeling physically unwell, as if dragged through razor blades, I put the curled bill down.

With McD's parents' check we had acquired a four-room railroad apartment on the corner of Avenue A and Houston, right across from Katz's Deli and Jasper Johns's old studio.

We moved in and had an iron bed that the three of us slept in and a green velvet armchair that David had found in the trash. A friend gave us a white cat that McD christened Puff (after the Dick-and-Jane books) to catch the many mice. But Walter and David kept fighting, and finally Walter moved out. He had his mail delivered to our mailbox, and one day a check came from his unemployment. McD took it to the bank and cashed it. Another huge fight ensued when Walter came to collect his mail. Many "Fuck you"s were exchanged as Walter left.

Back in the downtown scene, we heard a lot about Keith Haring's and Jean-Michel Basquiat's increasing fame. In the year we were away they were the young artists progressing from shows at the Mudd Club and Club 57 to international exhibitions. In the 1980s the East Village was a place one moved to because of the cheap rent. McD's original apartment where he paid fifty dollars a month was on East Third across from a men's shelter which is still there. Punks, writers, painters, filmmakers, drag queens all mixed with the local Polish and Hispanic population. The Bowery was a place with SRO hotels, Christian missions for the homeless, addicts, and drunks. The streets were filthy with garbage; men were passed out lying on the sidewalks' warm grilles; there were human feces everywhere and many rats scurrying about the decrepit buildings. When we walked around, McD liked to point out the early-nineteenth-century buildings and the old bars from a time when the Bowery was as desirable as Fifth Avenue as a place to live. Below Houston Street was another world from the East Village where there were old shops, some open but many closed. It looked like a ghost town at night. Chrystie Street, along Roosevelt Park, was lined with prostitutes in high platform boots and miniskirts.

When we didn't have a penny, we'd go visiting. We'd walk around town and visit David's friends to see who might be home, ring the bell, and hope that they'd offer some coffee and toast and maybe an egg. Lunch was tougher as most people worked.

When we were truly desperate and starving and not one bell was answered, we found AA meetings where they served coffee and cookies and occasionally cake. We'd wait and quietly come in late, then sit in the back and get a plateful of cookies and a coffee. We liked the dramatic stories that the people in front would tell. Some were funny, others tragic, but there was a comforting sobriety at the end. "It's kind of like an MGM movie," McD would say, "because there's always a happy ending." One day a skinny old leftie queen approached us. "What are you doing here?" I feared we were caught. McDermott blurted out, "I'm addicted." Eyebrows were raised. "To the meetings," he said as we walked out. We stopped going to that meeting, but there were plenty more.

There was one old-fashioned restaurant in Little Italy named Luna. Its interior was still intact from the past, with old paintings and furniture. But for us to sit and have dinner would be too costly. So I'd walk over and get takeout. We shared the five-dollar container of soft spaghetti with a glob of marinara sauce and three large, overcooked meatballs. I'd place it on two of the few chipped Victorian plates we had and fill our tumblers with grape juice. We'd each get one meatball and then split the last. While I waited for the meal, I had a perfect view of a tall monster of a man with a *Texas Chainsaw Massacre* kind of look, who washed the dishes. When the waiter brought the finished plates in to be washed, he'd take food off, gobbling the good parts that were left as he threw the dish into the large sink below.

Unlike Jean-Michel and Keith, most of our lot were barely making ends meet. Filmmaker Eric Mitchell, who lived above musician John Lurie of the Lounge Lizards, was still in David's old building on East Third. Eric or John, I don't remember which, would run an electric extension cord down from a window to get electricity from whoever had it when he couldn't pay the bill.

David heard Justin had moved to the city just a block from our Avenue A apartment. We found the address and rang the bell. A dark-haired, very good-looking fellow asked us in after telling us Justin was upstate. His name was John Patrick Fleming. He showed us some photographs, and in one he had a Mohawk haircut and in another he was perform-ing a whip dance in San Francisco. Patrick, as he was called, told us he was thirteen when he first met a sixteen-year-old Justin, who was passed out in a snowbank. We told Walter we found him a boyfriend with the same last name; then David put them together. At first Patrick was noncommittal, and we had to console Walter. McD said to him, "It's difficult to tame a wild animal." But they soon became a couple.

Patrick found me a job selling gourmet sandwiches in a wicker bas-ket door-to-door in the Seventh Avenue fashion district. Patrick and one of his friends made the sandwiches. I'd wait on Seventh Avenue until a white van pulled up and I'd get inside with a few other des-perate characters and be given my gingham-lined basket and a list of what sandwiches were in it. Then I'd go into a building floor-to-floor and door-to-door. "Ding dong, Avon calling," I kept repeating to myself. I was back on my old fashion-job stomping grounds, but in a not-so-glamorous way. One woman asked me if I was Peter from FIT. Like the apostle Peter, I denied it.

At first I made a lot of money, seventy dollars a day. McD knew what

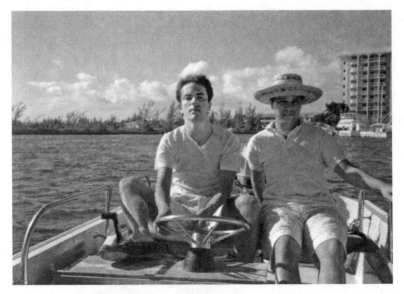

John Patrick Fleming and Walter Fleming

time I got off and we would have any extra sandwiches for dinner and spend the money on a movie, some antique or other, get our clothes out of hock at the dry cleaner's or his silver pocket watch from a pawnshop. In the morning I'd have just enough left for the seventy-five-cent subway fare and my dollar coffee-and-donut breakfast at Chock Full o'Nuts.

Soon the customers got tired of the sandwiches—day after day of the same chicken salad or salami-and-sprouts. We were sick of them, too. So the money dwindled weekly, till all I made was twenty dollars a day.

"This is ridiculous," David protested. "We're artists, not salesmen. And you only bring home a little bit now. We have paintings to finish."

"But what about money? We never have any," I cried in vain.

"We're not going to get rich and famous by selling sandwiches. You'll have to quit." I agreed and let Patrick know.

Cookie Mueller told me how she had had a job at a collection agency and had to call and threaten people to pay their bills. She wasn't that kind of person at all. One of the coolest people around, she also wrote the greatest stories. Cookie hated that job, the people there, and what was required of her. She then took all the names on her list, called all the people personally, and told them she destroyed their reports and that they would never have another threatening call.

We convinced ourselves that artists don't take full-time jobs. David would get some singing gigs at the Pyramid Club or I'd get a job with a decorator to do some stenciling. Once we didn't eat for two days. We were very thin. If we had five dollars, we could either go to the Kiev, a Polish restaurant on Second Avenue, where for a fiver we could get two bowls of soup and a large side of challah bread. Or we could wait and go to bed hungry and get two full breakfasts and a bottomless cup of coffee at 103 Second, a twenty-four-hour modern diner a block from the Kiev.

For some extra cash I sold my beloved pink suit and other clothes to a black rockabilly singer I knew from the club scene. We still had two sets of dress shoes from Brooks Brothers. Also, the two 1930s rayon suits, a navy double-breasted and a single-breasted in brown. Over time and with much wear, they became shiny, wrinkled, and frayed. But that added to our "shabby genteel" look.

One day on our rounds we were headed to Roseanne's loft in Tribeca. We were on the street in SoHo, fighting, and as I was blaming David for ruining my life, walking across West Broadway, I heard a voice call out, "Excuse me, may I take your picture?" I turned and saw a curly-headed young woman. I yelled, "*No!* Get away from us."

David cooed back, "Of course you can take our picture. Peter, how can you be so rude?"

We later saw the picture in *The Village Voice*. I was frowning. The photographer was Amy Arbus, daughter of Diane Arbus. She was photographing people's street fashion, which ended up being mostly our friends from the East Village. The image later ended up in a 1983 *L'Uomo Vogue* magazine, showing the trends in fashion, and our look was considered the look of the following year. Except our look was vintage rags.

When we got especially desperate, we would visit Vivian, who worked at the General Motors Building on Fifth Avenue between Fifty-Eighth and Fifty-Ninth. Since we didn't have money for the subway, we'd take a long walk uptown. In any case, in the summer the trains were unbearably hot, with the only breeze from open windows and ceiling fans that felt like a blow dryer had been turned on you. And some car windows were so covered with graffiti that we couldn't see what station it was. On our walks we'd always stop off at the main library on Forty-Second Street to look at *Kindred Spirits* by Asher B. Durand, a painter of the Hudson River School, which depicts the artist Thomas Cole and the poet William Cullen Bryant standing on a rocky ledge overlooking the Catskills. (The library later sold it for forty million dollars to Alice Walton for her Crystal Bridges Museum.) McD would entertain me with stories of his past to kill time on the way.

We finally reached the destination in Midtown. If we didn't have the dime to call his mother, David would go upstairs and come back with her. She'd sometimes walk with us around the block to hear what we were doing and give us some cash and encouragement. Vivian believed in her son's talent. She would give him a talking to and advise him to "use all your talents" and get to work and make some money. He'd nod his head and say his goodbyes when she handed him cash. Once he walked away in a huff from some advice she'd given him. She handed me some bills and said, "I wasn't prepared for a child like him."

It was fair to say that everything was secondary to David's passion for living in his "time machine." He told me that from age fourteen he'd made a conscious decision to dress in the past; he considered the interiors he created to be his greatest artwork, and felt that one day he would disappear into the past. I accepted that. He seemed to know everything. He showed me the differences between the centuries through antique furniture, high and low, from dress to interiors, then manners, even letter writing. For him, everything modern was disposable. His past was about permanence. "They made it to last!" he'd shout. "Now it's all plastic consumerist culture!"

McD would tell me stories of his youth. He moved to New York without finishing his last year at Syracuse University because he met Richard Merkin, a visiting artist. Richard was an immaculately dressed straight man costumed in the *Esquire* thirties style of bowler hats and walking sticks. Merkin and McD had a lunch of a hot-dog-and-Brussels-sprout casserole in McD's off-campus apartment in a poor neighborhood of Syracuse, which he had decorated with antiques from the street ("Nobody wanted old things then") and bright pink walls (because "that was the color the landlord gave me"). Afterwards, Merkin pulled McD aside and said, "You could be the greatest eccentric in Syracuse and no one would ever hear of you in Utica. You have to move to New York."

McD took his advice, quit school—much to his mother's annoyance—and left for Manhattan. He rented one room on the Upper West Side, on Eighty-Second Street just off Central Park, which eventually led to him renting the whole floor and then later the floor above. McD restored the rooms to their original 1880s grandeur. Then he convinced his college friends in Syracuse to move to New York and start an art salon. His landlady was Janet Jacob Adams, an old society matron down on her luck. He said she had a Sargent portrait above the fireplace.

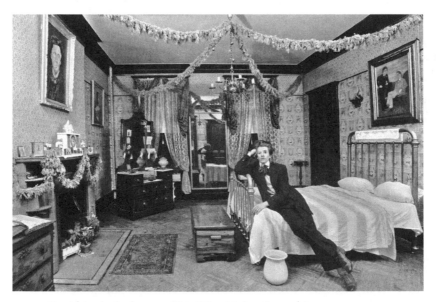

David in the bedroom of his West Eighty-Second Street apartment

A painting professor at Syracuse, Jerome Witkin, photographer Joel Peter Witkin's twin brother, made a portrait of McD sitting on top of the Empire State Building. "I'll pay you to sit," he said.

"I don't want any money. I'm moving to New York and I want a letter of introduction."

Witkin gave him the promised letter and a list of names to call upon. On the list were painter Alice Neel, Jean-Paul Goude (then *Esquire*'s art director, and later Grace Jones's art director and lover), writer Glenn O'Brien, and *Saturday Night Live* head writer Michael O'Donoghue, among others.

After he stripped the paint off the baseboards and doorframes, he put up vintage flowered wallpaper, started to entertain, and handed out his folded mimeographed magazine, of which there was only one issue, *The Cottage: Protector of Hearth and Home.* Janet Jacob Adams was a friend of Philip Van Rensselaer, the aristocratic socialite and author of several books, including a memoir called *Rich Was Better.* David invited him for tea upstairs. Philip loved McD's place but said the chandelier was "very white trash" and had to go.

Since McD liked to entertain, he was planning a Grand Ball in his apartment; he had Tiffany-engraved invitations sent out. One he posted to the couturier Charles James who had burnt many bridges in the fashion industry and was living in poverty at the Chelsea Hotel. I used to see him when I lived at the hotel for a month in the late seventies, but we never spoke. In a few days McD received a missive from Mr. James. In his letter Mr. James stated how ridiculous it was to have a Grand Ball in the late afternoon. "And what would one wear?" he wrote. "Morning dress, to a Grand Ball? Or white tie in the afternoon?" He declined the invitation.

During his bank-messenger days McD had to deliver an envelope to Hope Hampton, the former silent-movie star. (The press dubbed her "Hopeless Hampton" for her lack of acting skills.) In preparation for delivering the letter, McD bought a 1920s *Photoplay* with her face on the cover. When he arrived, Miss Hampton descended the zebra-carpeted

stairs. He told the butler he had to give the bank envelope to her personally. He then handed her the old magazine.

"Look, I've brought you the latest issue of *Photoplay*. You're on the
cover!" he gleefully stated. Not knowing if he was making fun of her,
she took the magazine, and as she started to ascend the zebra-covered
staircase she paused and turned to slowly look at him. "Why don't you
get some new clothes? Your outfit is very out of date."

There is no question I was a bit mesmerized by McD, as despite all
the volatility and crazy theories, he was highly intelligent and liked
a serious conversation. All his quirks and oddities were so different
from mine. I was such an introvert and he was the premier extrovert.

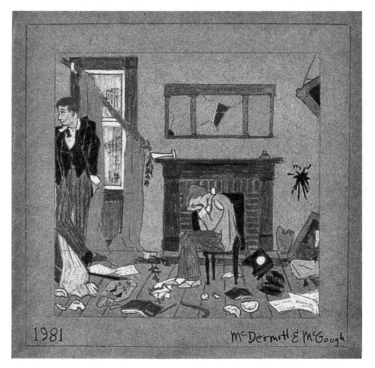

Saying no to McD meant overturned tables and smashed mirrors,
among other things.

His energy was boundless. I soon learned the hard way that "No" was not an answer he kindly took to. "No" led to overturned tables or a screaming match.

On our daily ritual of walking through different neighborhoods we often visited Edit DeAk in her SoHo loft on Wooster Street, with its many artists' graffiti tags and paintings by Basquiat and Francesco Clemente on the walls. Edit, who had escaped from Communist Hungary in the trunk of a car, was a brilliant art critic who wrote for *Artforum* and cofounded *Art-Rite* magazine with the "neopop" artist Walter Robinson. In one of her articles she wrote that artists were like Cabbage Patch Kids dolls, each with its own personality and papers, and suggested the magazine just print the artists' names in bold letters because that's all they were interested in—seeing their names. She told me David was a genius. There were three art critics/curators at that time who got a lot of attention: Edit, who introduced Clemente to New York in an *Artforum* article; Rene Ricard, poet, Warhol actor, critic, and artist, who wrote for *Artforum* a piece on Julian Schnabel ("Not about Julian Schnabel") and one on Haring and Basquiat ("The Radiant Child"); and Diego Cortez, aka Jimmy Curtis, who started the Mudd Club with Anya Phillips (the legendary downtown punk and Deborah Harry's best friend) and club owner Steve Mass. (Its original name was the Molotov Cocktail Lounge.) Diego also curated the *New York/New Wave* show at PS1 (now part of MoMA) in Queens, of which Basquiat became the star. When McD took me to visit Anya Phillips, who also was a dominatrix, she had a white man wearing a maid's uniform cleaning her apartment. He paid her to clean it. When he came near the table where we were sitting, she kicked him with one of her stiletto heels and said, "Leave us, slave."

We also attended services at the Middle Collegiate Church, a Dutch Reformed church on lower Second Avenue with an intact period interior, including Tiffany stained-glass windows and gold-stenciled walls; but the clincher for us was the 1911 Edison electric cross of light bulbs

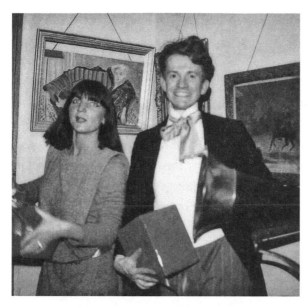

McD with Edit DeAk in the Avenue C apartment

above the altar. Every Thursday they gave a luncheon for the elderly ladies of the church, and the rotund church organist played old songs as the matronly ladies dined at several long tables covered with paper tablecloths. The organist told us that as a youth he was at the famous Minsky's burlesque house, playing piano for the strippers, when it was raided and shut down. We were there most weeks to ease ourselves into the luncheon. Since we attended weekly services (we didn't join the church, because that meant dues and fees), we felt it would be fine to create a studio in a large, windowed room below the minister's apartment. We gradually brought in an easel, some canvases, and paint and set up a corner sharing the room with a boys' karate class. McD was moving antique furniture from the attic and basement of the church to furnish our studio. "Well, they're not using them!" he reprimanded me when I protested. From an old store on the Lower East Side we bought three large rose-flowered linoleum carpets from the forties that were still in stock. The minister wanted a younger congregation, and we felt comfortable with the white-haired members.

David was generous but often lacked normal people skills. He would say whatever popped into his head with no filter: "You look so fat," or "You got old." Most people were really put off by his comments. I had found a book from 1928 called *The Game of Life and How to Play It* by Florence Scovel-Shinn; her husband was Everett Shinn, the Ashcan School painter. The book, a version of *The Power of Positive Thinking*, was about silent films, crank Victrolas, and double-decker buses. She wrote sentences like, "My ship comes in over a calm sea," and "All things I seek are now seeking me." She called this thinking "Divine Mind." McD loved the old-fashioned rhetoric. I finally had a control button. If he went into a rage or was just about to say something that would offend someone, I'd say, "That's not Divine Mind." He'd quickly stop his rant and become nice.

One day, walking up Second Avenue, we ran into Maripol, who let us know in her French accent, "David, Jean-Paul Goude is looking for you. He wants you for an Orangina commercial. Give him a call." Goude answered and said he already had cast the part, but to come over anyway. We went to his apartment on Union Square and he did a video of McD in a waiter's uniform. They sent the film to Paris and McD got the job. The commercial was shot in Florida to look like the French Riviera. We not only arranged for two tickets, but David wanted a third for his latest crush, a cute straight French boy whose mother owned a little bistro on Fifth Street. Maripol did the costumes for the commercial and kept teasing David's new crush.

The French boy paid for the taxi to the airport and off we went. When we arrived, they put us in a fancy modern hotel in Miami. McD immediately hated it and managed to get hold of the week's rent. With the wad of cash they gave him, he moved us into a seedy 1930s hotel that looked like where Lana Turner might have drunk herself to death in some B movie. They dyed McD's hair an even brighter shade of red and glued a tray with soda bottles to his hand. He played a waiter with a tray of drinks that customers were chasing him for as he slid down a water slide. The hip-hop dancer kid they hired from the Bronx who was supposed to fly down the water slide and do flips got the flu. So David took it all on, the slide as well as doing flips over and over again,

into the pool's cold water. Jean-Paul congratulated him on his profes-
sionalism and said he could become a big star. The producers forgot to
have him sign the contracts, and when they did come by, he refused.

"Forget it! No way. With all the work I had to do? I want more
money. You people just want to kill me!"

They did now. One woman yelled at him and said, "You'll never
work in show business again!" and McD retorted loudly, "Well, if it
saves me from ever having to see you again, that's just fine!"

They came back in an hour with seven thousand dollars in cash and
a blank contract. We had never seen that kind of money. He looked
at me and I nodded yes to take it. David signed the carte blanche
after I counted the money three times. It felt very underworld and
show-business as I took the money and practically pinned it to my
underwear.

We bade our goodbyes and found a hotel to move into that was right
out of the movie *La Cage aux Folles*. I think it was last decorated in the
fifties. The lobby was filled with nude male bronzes and fake rococo
furniture that looked like what you would find in the furniture stores in
Little Italy. The owners were a couple of queens who you could tell had
been together for decades. A thin, dyed-blond man with a withering
mustache was at the reception desk and was thrilled to be paid in cash.

"My, such young, clean-looking fellows with so much cash!" he said
as he looked into the envelope.

"Oh, Mary, please, leave these children alone!" cried his barrel-chested
partner, the "chicken" of the couple. He had a jet-black pompadour (a
toupee, for sure) and a red silk shirt open to the waist to show his hairy
and very tan chest, with strings of gold chains to match the many rings
that sparkled as he held out a tumbler of vodka with a splash of cran-
berry. The ice cubes chimed against the glass as his arms waved about.

"These kids want to get to their room—all three of them!" He
winked.

We all—including the French crush—crammed into a tiny elevator
with our host and luggage. He opened the door to another gay time
machine from the fifties. It had plush velvet bedspreads and matching

window drapery, a tiny crystal chandelier, and two stools made to look like Roman camp chairs with swords as legs, and beds to match. The host flopped into an armchair, looking ready to grow roots. "I hope you boys will be comfortable. Everyone's very friendly here." His tone suddenly became rather wanton. We just stood there in silence until he got the hint and jumped up and spilled some of his drink, rubbing it into the carpet with his loafer. "Oopsie!" he said, departing.

At the end of our Florida travels we said goodbye to our French friend who didn't want to stay with us, so we sent him in a taxi to the airport back to New York.

"Why don't we take a train to Williamsburg, Virginia, and then go see Nana?" David cried. Nana had moved from New Jersey to her birthplace, Raleigh, North Carolina, and bought a "McMansion" and a new Cadillac.

"But we have free plane tickets to New York," I complained.

"Who cares? Planes are horrible. It's like a bus with wings. And we'll have a sleeping compartment." He was right. The train room was nice, and we could sit or lie down and look out at the passing landscape. This is when the dining cars on trains had linen tablecloths, silverware, and a bud vase on the table.

We put some cash into two money orders after we booked our train tickets to Virginia. One for all the many months of rent we owed Kristian and one for when we returned to New York for other bills. The rest was for our trip. On our arrival we stayed in the Williamsburg Hotel and ate in luxury and rambled about the re-created eighteenth-century town, picking up decorating tips for the future. We met a wig maker there who said she could make our hair into eighteenth-century wigs. We left with a few souvenirs and headed to Raleigh.

When we arrived at Nana's newly built home, we couldn't believe how ugly it was. Nana was in an excited frenzy to see us. "What do you think of my new house? Don't I look rich?" Nana asked happily. I kept silent. Inside was all the furniture from New Jersey and a brand-new color TV console. "Look how big the TV is!"

We were shown our room. It was furnished from her early poor

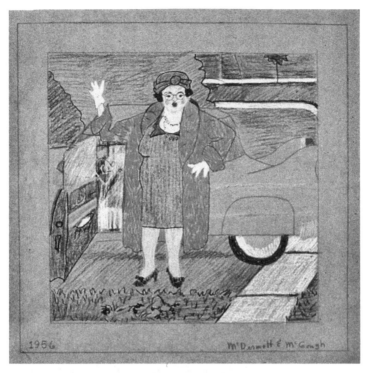

Nana, McD's granny, with pink Cadillac c. 1956

days with a vanity table made out of crates covered in frilly fabric. The art consisted of a paper plate turned around with a cut-out picture of Shirley Temple held to the wall by ribbon and a pushpin. Later, in the early nineties, we would make a series of art based on that room for a show in Paris. Nana showed us the surveillance camera she had in her front window. It was a square tissue box and a cut toilet-paper roll glued together and painted black. "Just to fool them. Locks are made for honest people, to keep them honest." She had a delicious meal of fried chicken, collard greens, and black-eyed peas set out on the table for us, with homemade coconut cake, ice cream, and coffee. Nana loved to watch C-SPAN, so afterwards we watched the news. She was a Baptist and completely right-wing, except she was for gay rights because of her adored, and only, grandson.

"I told my minister when he wanted me to sign a petition against homosexuals that they were born that way. It's a scientific fact. Well, he didn't like that at all!"

Nana was getting to me, in a good way. On the news was a black minister accused of beating a child in his congregation to death with a stick. Nana stood up in front of the television, pointing to the preacher on the screen, and screamed, "You dirty bastard! Beatin' and killin' a poor little child like that! Killin' a poor innocent baby. Someone should take a stick and beat you to death. That poor little child, it's terrible." I could sense this was bringing up some old trauma of hers. The minister continued trying to skirt the situation, saying, "The real problem here is integration." Then Nana's head started to bob, and she started to get excited. "That's right! He's right, it's integration! That's the problem. The birdies don't mingle. You don't see a robin a goin' with a blue jay."

David interrupted her rant. "Nana, Nana, we're going to bed."

"Well . . ." She paused and looked at me, worried I might judge her. "He still should be beaten for killing a poor little baby like that. It's a real, real shame . . . hurting an innocent child." Her head shook a bit, and she was talking and humming to herself. She called down the hallway, "I'll have breakfast in the morning."

We didn't have much cash on us, so David asked Nana after breakfast if she could cash the smaller money order. She stared at us and flew into a rage as if a demon had possessed her. "You came down here to rob me!" Her eyes were wide, and she was trembling. David tried to reason with her. "Nana, it's a money order. It's not a check. The money is there."

"Well, I'm not a bank!" She went on about how we were trying to get the money from her and cheat her. At that McD burst out, "We're leaving! Come on, Peter—let's go." We threw our belongings into a suitcase and left the room. At that, Nana started to cry out and beg him to stay. I did feel sorry for her just then.

But David was furious now, and he started to scream. "We made a special trip to visit you, and you just made a big fight thinking we're going to rob you! How ridiculous is that? I have my own money now!" His voice echoed through her cathedral-like ceiling. As we neared the front door, she held on to his arm and begged him to stay. I didn't want to get in the middle of it or have anyone's rage turn on me. We left her house and started walking through the tree-lined suburban neighborhood to the train station. After a few blocks we heard Nana calling out, "David! David!" We turned and saw her in the new Cadillac. She was wearing an old raincoat and had put on a turban. Gone were her cat-eyed glasses, replaced by large new ones. She called out, "I'll cash your check! Please come back, honey!"

"Forget it!" David screamed. "I don't want your lousy money!" She drove on.

We walked to the train station and found her there waiting. We waited with the other passengers as they watched this drama unfold. She kept begging him to come back, right up until the train arrived. I felt sorry for her. I had rarely experienced fighting in my family. We kept our rage inside. Once back in New York, after paying our long-overdue bills, added to our expenses from the trip, what was left from the seven thousand was two hundred dollars. Broke again, I picked up *The Game of Life* and started rereading it.

9

Around this time, we met a taxi driver named Ricky Clifton. Ricky had three favorite subjects at the time: Japan, where he had studied ikebana (Ricky's flower arrangements are beautiful) and ceramics; Tina Chow (for her birthday he went to Chinatown and bought a big white porcelain Buddha and took it to Warhol and had him write his signature all over it); and opera. Ricky loved opera and would always know which production was the best and who were the greatest singers. He worshiped Maria Callas.

We went to the opera with Ricky many times, and one cold autumn evening he said, "Meet me out front of the Met—I'll get the tickets." We arrived duded up in full-dress tails, capes, and top hats. The tickets were for standing room.

"What! Standing room?" we exclaimed.

"Just relax!" Ricky advised us. "You wait until just before the opera starts and then run into empty seats." Immediately he disappeared ahead of us into the theater. McD and I tried it, but we were caught and asked to leave. Once outside, we saw we had more than two hours to kill, so we took a walk and found ourselves in Times Square. We saw an old theater, the Adonis, playing gay porn, and decided to go in to get out of the cold. The lobby was still intact and beautiful, with

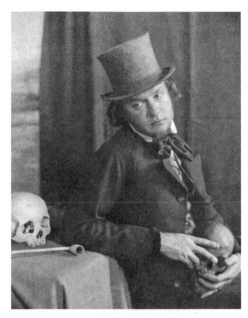

Our portrait of Ricky
for his birthday

etched glass chandeliers; so we went inside to sit, watched the movie, and left to make our way back to Lincoln Center.

Ricky also had the reputation of being a party crasher. Ricky didn't need an invitation—if he wanted to go, he went. This was confirmed in Bob Colacello's book *OUT* where the caption under Ricky's picture is "Party Crasher." Ricky knew everyone in the art world and showed up at most openings and dinners. At that time, Ricky was living in a long, slim storefront on Sixth Avenue and Prince Street. He decorated it to look like a traditional Japanese interior. The front was a gallery, and behind a curtain in the back was a futon. When we met him, he had a Christmas-ornament show displayed on a small Christmas tree in the window. He asked different artists like Warhol and Basquiat to paint a bulb. We begged him to let us make one. So we wrote on ours "Merry Christmas, Holly Solomon," for the SoHo art dealer we were courting. We asked Ricky for a show and we said we would make Meiji-period paintings, that moment when Japan allowed Western culture and trade in. Of course, Ricky loved the idea.

We found our stretchers in the trash, pulled them apart, and then bought ten-inch stretcher bars and made long canvases. McD explained that he was always looking to do the opposite of what others were doing. We found a book on traditional Japanese prints and changed the kimonos to suits and bustle dresses.

One day, on Houston Street, we ran into a young fellow from Italy named Massimo Audiello. At the time he was Diego Cortez's boyfriend. We were carrying all the little genre paintings we had just made. McD wanted to take them around and sell them to our rich friends which really just meant anyone who had a job. David laid the paintings out on the sidewalk to show them to Massimo.

"Oh, that's nice! . . . Oh, yes . . . Very funny!" he exclaimed after each one was placed strategically. "How much?"

David pointed to each one on the pavement. "This is seventy-five dollars. This one is fifty, this one hundred, and this one is one hundred and twenty-five. Which one do you want to buy?"

"Oh, I don't have any money!" Massimo exclaimed, laughing, in his thick Italian accent. David immediately picked up the canvases and bade him goodbye. We eventually sold most of them and made around three hundred dollars.

Diego Cortez had come to our studio in 1983 when it was in the basement of the Middle Collegiate Church on Second Avenue, and David made a drawing of him which years later I heard he had torn up. It did look like a kid's rendition of an old post-office Wanted sign. Within a month, we moved upstairs in the church's sunlit studio making fifteen paintings for Ricky's show. Diego came back and proposed that he be our agent. We were thrilled, because he had been Basquiat's and Haring's agent. He asked us if we were going to run out of ideas. I thought that was the craziest question. I've always had so many ideas, though some artists can make a career with just one idea and repeat it over and over again. Art is about ideas. In the 1980s Warhol was asking people for ideas. I had an assistant recently who worked for a young, hip artist who had a piece of paper on the wall that read "Ideas," and he asked the assistants to write down any he could use.

For the invitation to our show in the spring of 1983, Ricky made out

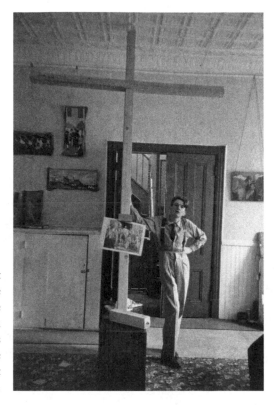

David in the studio at the Middle Collegiate Church on Second Avenue and Seventh Street, with New Amsterdam paintings on the wall. We made the cross for the Bleecker Street gallery's exhibition.

of an eraser a stamp of cherry blossoms, which he imprinted on each invitation in pink ink. One of Diego's clients purchased half the show, and an Italian gallerist, Lucio Amelio, wanted the remaining works held for consideration. Ricky took a painting of a young man cutting cherry blossoms as payment for having the show. Diego continued to bring clients to the studio, but we didn't produce as fast as his former artists.

Before Diego started working with us, we had met a young artist from Israel, Izhar Patkin, who lived next door to Edit. Izhar had asked David to perform for the opening of his show at Holly Solomon's gallery at 392 West Broadway. First he sang Grandmaster Flash's "The Message," rewritten by David to be more old-fashioned, accompanied by a quartet, a piano, a violin, and a horn while a female contortionist dressed as a bride bent over a grand piano, and then he sang our friend

Kristian's song "I Do," which later was made into a record. No one was paid, though Izhar suggested to Holly that she should visit our studio, and so we invited her to our apartment on Avenue A for tea. Walter, who was living with us at the time, played the butler and served us tea with finger sandwiches in our three-hundred-dollar-a-month tenement slum. We didn't have any paintings to show Holly. The few we had made in Hudson had sold for two hundred each, which we were thrilled to get. We borrowed a painting of Oscar Wilde that McD had done in the seventies from Glenn O'Brien; otherwise there were just blank canvases and a box of 1940s oil paints (hard as a rock) we had found lying around in the garbage. Holly commissioned a large portrait of herself for a frame that we had also found in the trash. We felt that maybe we were on our way.

Holly was an actress in her early life and then married Horace Solomon, whose family fortune was rumored to be from the invention of the plastic curler or the bobby pin. Anyway, Holly became a collector of pop art and had her portraits done by Lichtenstein and Warhol. In

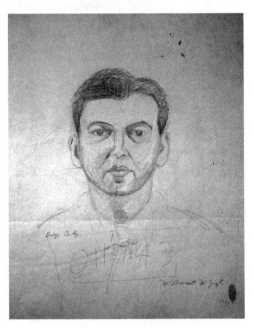

David's drawing of Diego Cortez

1969 she opened her own gallery at 98 Greene Street—becoming one of the first and one of the very few women gallery owners in SoHo, though Paula Cooper had opened her first gallery in 1968. We met Holly when she had her next gallery, on West Broadway, known for showing a movement called Pattern and Decoration. In 1978, a young gallerist named Mary Boone moved across the street from 420 West Broadway and stole the limelight from Holly, showing up-and-coming young artists like Julian Schnabel, David Salle, and Eric Fischl.

With the din of traffic and blasting music from Houston Street, Holly ascended the slanting steps into our apartment that had an old stove and a claw-foot bathtub in the entrance. The floors were so slanted that if you dropped a pencil it would roll across the room. Holly couldn't have been more charming. We were excited to have an actual art dealer visit. After tea was over and we made the deal, Holly exclaimed, "Let's have lunch!" We were thrilled. "Finally," I thought, one of the good restaurants in SoHo we couldn't afford. "Let's go to Katz's," she said. Katz's is a great-looking Jewish deli on Houston Street from before the forties. Their slogan, dating from World War II, is "Send a Salami to Your Boy in the Army," and a sign to that effect is still in the window. Disappointed as we were, we were happy to eat out. Holly paid two thousand dollars for the portrait, a huge sum for us. Izhar later told me one night at the Pyramid Club on Avenue A that it was a lot of money for anyone to get. We based the portrait on an eighteenth-century painting by the English artist George Romney and popped Holly's head on it. McD painted clipper ships in the East River as background. David's mother saw the portrait and exclaimed, "She looks bitter!"

When David's mother had given us the deposit for the four-room apartment, I thought, "How will we ever afford three hundred dollars a month?" But then suddenly McD wanted more apartments in the building. So, he took over one from a young poet and then another from a family, both directly below us. The one that belonged to the family had dog food littered around the kitchen corners, and a dog chain was screwed into the wooden fireplace mantel. The walls were filthy and cracked; holes in the plaster ceiling showed the wooden lath underneath; the tub and the stove were caked with grime; and there was a rats' nest under a counter. I was upstairs one day when I heard David scream. I thought he had found a stash of money. After I rushed downstairs, he said a huge rat had jumped out of a cardboard box he was filling with the debris and ran across his shoulder and out the door.

Whenever we bought groceries, McD would remove all the plastic and Styrofoam they were packed in and empty the contents into cookie jars or a fruit bowl and take the plastic to a recycling center. If he bought talcum powder, he'd empty it into a vintage glass bottle. After taking the modern labels off the canned food, we had a hard time figuring out what was in which can. In the morning, he'd pull the elastic thread from his socks and wear garters to hold them up. He found an old Jewish merchant on lower Tenth Avenue who could supply him with vintage drawstring underwear; he didn't care if it was stained from years of dust sitting on a shelf. He also had discovered a shop down near Wall Street, the Collar and Cuff Replacement Company, where he could bring new or used shirts and have them made into collarless shirts for detachable collars. He once had the tailor there make six shirts for us, three for him and three for me, but McD insisted that the tailor make them long like a nightshirt, so the French-cuffed sleeves hung below our fingers and we could use arm garters to hold them up.

We could hardly afford the three hundred a month for the rent let alone what would be a total of nine hundred for the three apartments he was planning on taking over. As a result, the electricity bill wasn't paid. No electricity meant living with candles, and our old brass fan couldn't work, so we only had hand-held ones. When it was hot outside it was *very* hot inside. One boiling day we came home, and the candles were bent over like dead tulips. We'd be sweating at night and David would announce, "I'm impervious to the heat," but he would run the tub and take a lukewarm bath before bed, leaving the tub full to take cool dips throughout the night. He'd insist on keeping all the windows and the door to the apartment open to get cross ventilation. One night a man from the street came to our open door. David heard something and walked to the door with a lit candle glowing against his white nightshirt. The man shrieked as though seeing an apparition of Wee Willie Winkie and apologized, "Sorry, lady," as he ran down the stairs.

In some ways our slum tenement home on Avenue A was comforting and transporting. McD would pick up large potted plants off the street and nurse them back to health. As always, our furniture also came from the street. He picked up every chair he thought worthy. One afternoon a young woman came to visit us for tea, and we sat around the fire reading my father's copy of *Alice in Wonderland*. As the gloaming approached, we lit the candles as we continued reading aloud. I must say it was truly enchanting—so much so, the young woman seemed to turn into a little girl before my eyes. I thought she was going to dissolve in tears. It was a place out of time. It could have easily been 1883.

One day a college friend of David's, the photographer Josef Astor, invited us to an afternoon party. Josef was staying at an apartment David had helped decorate and had lived in until he was thrown out. McD constantly lost apartments. The Ageloff Tower was built in 1929 at 141 East Third Street to keep the neighborhood Jews from moving to the suburbs. It was nicknamed "the Jewish Splendor." Josef's roommate's apartment, on the top floor with views of the East River, was decorated in period furniture, down to the old refrigerator with a circular motor on top.

In the large dining room a group of confirmed bachelors stood around a table with cakes and tea sandwiches on colored Fiestaware platters while 1930s dance music played in the background. At the height of the party Andy Warhol arrived with his sidekick photographer Christopher Makos and some more bachelors. All conversation stopped. The only sound was the crooner on the stereo. We couldn't believe it, and we all froze in silence. No one spoke or moved until Josef went over to him and Chris. As Andy crossed the room, everyone followed him into the dining room and watched as if it were a play.

After a lot of silence and staring, the room became more relaxed, and people started whispering to one another about Andy. Warhol was standing with Josef (they both were models for the Zoli Agency—another brilliant ploy of Andy's) against a sideboard, chatting and looking over the remains of cakes and sandwiches on the colorful dishes.

I watched as McD, in a very blasé way, positioned himself next to his college pal Josef and Andy to become part of the conversation. They shook hands as David was introduced, and chatted too far from me to hear what was being said. Minutes later Andy left. I went over to David and asked what he had said to him.

"He was kind of quiet, but now I can say I met Andy Warhol." When McD first moved to New York, he told me, the two people he most wanted to meet were Truman Capote and Andy Warhol.

When David and I were living on the Bowery just above China-town and had only five dollars for dinner, we would often walk over to Tribeca to an Asian fish-fry restaurant across the street from the Odeon, a hip art-world, fashion, and movie crowd hangout, and share a plate of fried fish, French fries, and a can of soda while we looked out the window as the limousines pulled up across the street.

One night, Diego invited us to a Mary Boone dinner at the Odeon after the opening of her show for the German artist Markus Lüpertz.

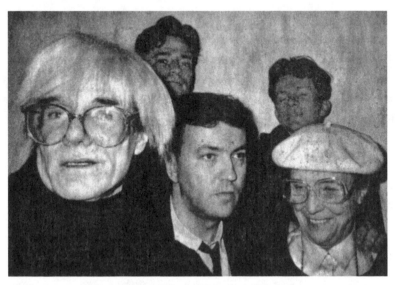

At the Robert Miller Gallery, left to right: Andy Warhol, me, Diego Cortez, McD, and Louise Bourgeois

David was seated at Andy's table, and I sat at the next table. Toward the end of the dinner, Andy asked the unusually quiet David a question. That was all he needed. David once told me that his ploy was to let everyone else get talked out so that he could get all the attention later. He went on a rant about how the current popular movie *E.T.* was about a young boy and his erection. He had already discussed this with Edit.

"What?" Andy laughed.

"Well," David continued, "when E.T. gets excited his neck lengthens, and it's like a young boy having his first experience with his erection." The table burst into laughter.

Before leaving, Andy asked us to be in his magazine.

My table was much more subdued, so I went downstairs to the bathroom. In the small lounge Diego and Jean-Michel were smoking a joint. I sat down. Admittedly, I was a little nervous because Jean-Michel was so cool and very famous now. Jean was friendly and complimented me on a painting he saw of ours at the Clementes' and then started asking me about my clothes and my tall, starched detachable collar from 1900. Jean-Michel had great style even when he was sleeping on other people's sofas and couldn't afford to buy expensive suits. He handed me this large half-smoked joint. I could tell its potency by the aroma. And in my most ladylike manner I accepted the spliff: "Oh, yes, surely, of course, thank you," I muttered shyly.

This made the already high Diego burst into laughter and fall into hysterics. We passed around the joint. I consciously was trying not to inhale too much. I bade my adieus and ascended the stairs. Winded at the top, I realized just how strong the marijuana truly was. I could feel it in my feet. My eyes looked over the mass of late-night diners. The noise felt deafening and the room seemed to move in slow motion. Cautiously I maneuvered my way back to my table, which was finishing coffee and dessert. "Dessert?" I thought. "How long was I down there?"

I inhaled the warm chocolate cake into my mouth. People had left or had moved seats. Andy had left before I met him. I was moving my head trying to get David's attention. I was too high, and I wanted to leave. I saw him talking animatedly to his table, where everyone appeared to be held in rapt attention. I couldn't catch his eye. "Oh, that jerk!" I cursed. "I have to get out of here."

I was beginning to feel paranoid as well, but then a bearded artist, Gary Stephan, who now was seated next to me, turned to speak. He had a very large, smoldering, and quite smelly cigar in his hand. He was blowing the smoke above him and somehow the billows of smoke mesmerized me. I eyed the curving wave of the stinking cloud.

"You're a painter?" His voice echoed and reverberated. It sounded like we were in a tin can. I turned my gaze from the heavenly billows. I felt as if I were under warm water. I tilted my head and paused. "Ah . . . why, yesss," I hissed. My fingers fondled my artistic tie as I stared at a piece of chocolate stuck in his beard.

"Well?" He seemed annoyed. "What do they look like?"

In my hazy stupor I paused. "Well . . ." I paused again. "Well . . . um . . . they're really . . . very . . . pretty. Yes! Very, very pretty."

An eternity passed. He stared at me through the smelly clouds that engulfed us. "Hmmph," he snorted, and turned his back to me. Again I thought, "I've really got to get out of here." I rose and furiously went over to David's table and interrupted his conversation. "We have to go!" I blurted.

"What? No way!" he said, waving me off. "Go away."

I looked over to his dinner partner and forced a smile. I leaned into David's ear.

"We have to go now," I whispered harshly.

"Forget it," he whispered back.

"No! We have to go *now*!" I pulled on his arm. "Please!"

"But I haven't had my dessert yet."

"We're going!" I grabbed his dessert off the plate and put it in his napkin and pulled him out of his seat. Outside in the evening air he reprimanded me.

"What is wrong with you? I was having such a good time!"

"I'm sorry! I smoked a joint with Diego and Jean-Michel," I cried, "and I freaked out. It was so strong."

"Well, what did you do that for?"

"I didn't want to look like a square when they offered it to me."

"I based my whole life on looking like a square," he reprimanded me. "Where's my dessert?"

"Oh—I left it on the table."

"Peter! What a gyp."

When *Interview* magazine contacted us about a photographer, David insisted on them hiring his old friend Editta Sherman, also known as "the Duchess of Carnegie Hall." They had known each other in another life in the early seventies. Editta was a mad eccentric who had a large costume collection that she would wear around town, such as a 1930s monkey-hair coat or a swan-feathered muff with two heads. She had a big, beautiful photography studio facing north above Carnegie Hall, where she posed us beside a column with a Roman bust on top. She set us up in different poses, wheeled the large wooden camera toward us, cranking handles to get the right shot, then put in a large sheet of film, ducked under a black cloth, and yelled, "Stand still! No blinking! One . . . two . . . three. Got it!" Pictures of Elvis, Sinatra, and Julie Newmar, whom she had photographed with her large wooden camera, covered her walls. Short and plump, with a bubble of very dark curls surrounding her pale, wrinkled face, Editta was nearing eighty at the time, and she died at one hundred and one.

Upon our departure she was wildly complimenting David on the full-dress tail suit he wore. I wore something more rustic and corduroy. "Wait!" she ordered as she disappeared behind a curtain, returning with a long ebony walking stick with a large gold ornamental top of leaves wrapping around a mother-of-pearl inset. We gushed as she handed it to David. "Now you're complete!" she beamed as she took him in. "*But*—it's only a loan. Don't forget!"

One weekend Nana was visiting New Jersey from the South and called to say she was coming with Vivian to bring groceries to us. We flew downstairs and met her in her Cadillac. When she opened the trunk, it was packed with groceries. David held up two long plastic-wrapped loaves of bread. The label read "2 for 99 cents."

"What is this?" he screamed. "I don't eat this garbage!"—and threw them back into the trunk. He then pulled on my arm, saying, "I can't eat this shit!," and stormed upstairs. On the staircase I kept begging him to be nice and to take the food. A few minutes later I could hear Nana screaming "David! *Daaaaavid!*" through the hallway. She found our apartment because David was at the top of the stairs screaming back at her. She came inside, short of breath and fuming.

"You dirty bastard!" she yelled. "I brought you all that food and I was gonna give you some money!"

"I don't want your crappy food or your dirty old whore money!" he screamed. "Now get out of here!"

"I'm not going anywhere!" Nana rebuffed. She stood by the door with her hands on her hips and looked over the slum tenement with its tub and stove in the entrance. "Look at this dump! You're paying three hundred dollars to live in the slums and I pay the same money to live in luxury!"

I just stood there in horror witnessing yet another family feud. I knew better than to get in the middle of the insanity. From what McD told me, quarrels with Nana had been going on for decades. In the bathtub was gray water from the morning laundry. David picked up a chipped enamel pail, scooped up some water, and holding it in front of her screamed, "If you don't leave, I'm going to throw this dirty water at you, Nana! Now get out!" He was almost laughing.

"You wouldn't dare do that! Don't—you—dare!" her voice escalated.

"*Get out!*" David screamed. "Now get out, Nana!"

"I'm not goin' anywhere. Don't you dare speak to me like that!"

"I'm warning you, Nana!" He threw the water on the floor by her feet and it splashed against her stockings.

"AHHHHHHHHH!" She let out a scream like the Wicked Witch in *The Wizard of Oz.*

"NOW GET OUT!" David's voice echoed out the doorway.

"Don't bother—I'm leavin'!" She went to the door, paused, turned around, looked at us, and muttered, "Deadbeats!"

Now, with the three apartments on Avenue A, David wanted to rent the corner room at Bradley and Kristian's on the Bowery, where he was living when I met him, as our painting studio, which he did. With three apartments, a painting studio, and three employees helping David, Holly's two thousand dollars went quickly. Before we knew it, we were deep in debt to our Avenue A landlord, Mr. Gambetta, and living back at the Bowery studio on Grand Street. Kristian was briefly furious with us that we hadn't told him our plan, but soon forgave us.

Now we were back in one room that leaked from the roof, with our few possessions and all of our canvases, including the large one of Holly. When it rained we had to fill one side of the room with bowls and pots to catch it all. We slept again in the single brass bed with a toilet down the hall; the room had a sink that wasn't connected so we also had to empty that bucket. It seemed like the entire punk scene came through Kristian and Bradley's door. Some slept in a loft bed in the hallway, others on a sofa. They also had a basement that bands would rent to rehearse in. David knew Kristian early on from his appearance with Lance Loud in *An American Family*. Lance was the son who moved to the Chelsea Hotel and came out on TV.

Paul Bridgewater, now the owner of the Bridgewater Gallery in the East Village, brought over some clients with the publicist/art agent Anne Livet to the Bowery. We had about seven small paintings at different stages of completion. When the prospective buyers asked about one or another we said they weren't finished. They thanked us and left without buying anything. Furious with no sales, McD went to each painting and signed them, cursing the collectors. "Now they're finished!" he grumbled. Soon enough we did finish them all.

We were finishing Holly's portrait in the Bowery studio when McD had the idea of finishing it in Holly's gallery. "We need some new inspiration. It's too crowded here." It never occurred to David to ask anyone in the gallery first. I agreed, so we walked the large painting over to West Broadway, set it up in the back storage/showroom, leaning it against a wall, and sat on the floor to work on it. At first Holly didn't seem to mind. Then she brought in a client she knew who had an art-nouveau gallery uptown that showed Tiffany lamps and other high-end objects. Holly showed her the artists she was exhibiting. The woman came up to us and asked what we were doing. McD immediately stood at attention for an audience. He went on explaining his theories, like "all time exists at the same time," and why we painted Holly the way we did, placing her in eighteenth-century Manhattan with clipper ships in the background. After his lecture the woman turned to Holly. "Why aren't you showing *them*? This is much more interesting than what you've shown me today." I gritted my teeth. I didn't dare look at Holly and kept painting. But Holly was all smiles. They departed. We said our goodbyes. Five minutes later Holly came back, enraged.

"Take that painting and all your belongings and get out of here! I'm running a business. You've disrupted enough here today," she said, and turned on her heel. We quietly gathered our paints and brushes in the now hushed atmosphere of the gallery as we slithered by the front desk with downcast eyes. We carried the large painting back through SoHo to our slum on the Bowery. When we put the painting down I burst into tears. "We're ruined. Our career is over. That was such a stupid idea." McD, who is more intellectual than emotional, was rarely comforting. He was trying to figure out the why rather than the how. But this time he was quite nice.

We had met a photographer at a nightclub who wanted to take our portrait, so we walked up to the Olympic Tower, on Fifth between Fifty-First and Fifty-Second Streets, famous for, among other things, the designer Halston having his showroom there. He took our picture; they had no food but very strong espresso. After walking all the way back to our studio on Grand Street with empty stomachs, David flew into a caffeinated frenzy and kicked a painting of a boy on a fence and slashed another called *Lot Leaving Sodom and Gomorrah*.

I caught him just in time before he attacked Holly's portrait. I screamed at him to get out. After he left, I crumpled into a chair. He returned hours later lamenting his rage. I decided to keep the slash in the *Lot* painting. I felt it added something.

When we finished Holly's painting, David said, "Let's put some museum juice on it!"

"What's that?"

"We mix some yellow ocher in the varnish to make it look worn and old," he explained. He then mopped the tall canvas with the yellowed varnish before we set it in the frame and then carried it over to Holly's gallery where it dried.

At the time I knew nothing about the art world and its intricate workings of collectors, agents, private dealers, art advisors, art critics, and the fine art of schmoozing. Sometimes the work seemed secondary to the artist's seductive personality that gets him or her in the door. I call it "the Goldilocks effect": not too hot—not too cold—just right. Art can get dated or go out of fashion. Or it gets rediscovered after decades of being forgotten: figurative art, cartoon art, minimalism, abstraction, graffiti, realism, and on and on. The moneyed art world of the heady eighties was just starting in SoHo. Out of the mob of artists looking for fame and fortune, only a handful are remembered today.

With SoHo seemingly impenetrable and all abuzz with artists on the rise, galleries started to show up in East Village storefronts with names like Gracie Mansion, New Math, Vox Populi, 8BC (Eighth Street between Avenues B and C), Nature Morte, Hal Bromm, and Semaphore East.

Alphabet City in the eighties resembled Berlin after the Second World War: blocks of windowless buildings, burnt-out cars, and mounds of bricks blocking the sidewalks. The occupants were the people who wouldn't leave or couldn't afford to. There were old Polish couples and Latino families, drug dealers and users, and artists, all of whom valued the cheap rents.

One gallery that became very famous was Patti Astor's FUN Gallery (1981–85), two storefronts on East Tenth Street. She had started out with an earlier basement gallery with Bill Stelling where she had shown Kenny Scharf, who had named it FUN. Patti was an actress who had starred with McD—along with other punk musicians and artists in the East Village—in Super 8 films that had a cult following in the late seventies. Eric Mitchell's 1980 film *Underground U.S.A.,* starring Patti Astor as a fading movie star, had a line around the block at the midnight showing at the St. Marks Cinema. Other downtown films of that time included Amos Poe's *Unmade Beds* (1976), with Deborah Harry; and Jim Jarmusch's *Permanent Vacation* (1980). McD starred as Caligula in James Nares's *Rome '78* (he showed me a news clipping that stated he was a more convincing Caligula than John Hurt in *I, Claudius*) and as part of a Nazi spy ring in Anders Grafstrom's *The Long Island Four* (1980). Nares later told David that he was in Los Angeles after the film was shown and was supposed to meet with Paramount Pictures. They were interested in him and wanted to meet David. But he missed the meeting and couldn't get another.

Patti had also starred in Charlie Ahearn's 1983 film *Wild Style,* about graffiti and the new sound called hip-hop in the Bronx, with Grandmaster Flash, Fab 5 Freddy, Lee Quinones (the protagonist), and Glenn O'Brien. With her gallery she brought in graffiti art from the Bronx to the rising art world of the East Village. These two worlds came together in her East Tenth Street FUN Gallery, which showed such artists as Quinones, Dondi, Crash, Daze, Futura 2000, and Fab 5 Freddy along with Basquiat, Haring, and Scharf. An article about the gallery appeared in *Artforum,* written by Rene Ricard and illustrated with Patti's portrait by Jimmy De Sana. This brought even more established art collectors, hangers-on, and Yoko Ono. With the new sounds of rapping and scratching booming out of the gallery, Patti's openings spread into the streets, and the mob there often brought the police. Hip-hop was pulled into punk/new wave and different camps that mulled around at the same time. Amidst all this, we were dressed in our early-twentieth-century style of detachable collars and frock coats. Graffiti art became a rage. Kids from the Bronx started making huge amounts of money, but even that would soon change.

Since we didn't have a telephone, one day in 1983 in our church studio Holly showed up unannounced with her husband, Horace. Weeks before we had agreed to be represented by Diego Cortez, so we didn't want to see her, since the last time we did she threw us out of her gallery. She walked in with a brown bag of lichee nuts. She handed them to us and started looking over the paintings. As shocked as we were, we asked them to sit down. She looked over the paintings we were making and offered us representation.

"Well . . ." David paused. "We are working with Diego. He's our agent now."

"I'm not interested in working with Diego!" Holly snapped. "I don't go through anyone else." Like Horace, I sat there in silence.

Somehow Holly's conversation came around to Edit.

"She's always been a great supporter of ours," David replied.

Holly's voice rose. "So have I!"

There was another pause. "Uh-huh," David mumbled.

"'Uh-huh'!" Holly grimaced. "What do you mean, 'Uh-huh'? Didn't I buy you that plane ticket so you could go to Rotterdam with Edit?"

"Yes," David agreed.

"And didn't I buy two paintings, the one of the lovers and the other painting of a cow? Well, you said it was a cow." (It was a pretty bad rendition of a cow.)

"Yes," David replied.

"And of course, there's my portrait," she added. That was a sore subject for me. "Well, then, what's the problem?" Holly asked.

"You dropped us, Holly," David hesitantly continued. "We wanted so badly to show with you and you just dropped us."

"I didn't drop anyone! You brought my portrait to the gallery to paint it! I'm running a business!" She kept shouting; I couldn't believe her anger.

"And now we're working with Diego. He's our agent," David repeated.

"Well, congratulations!" she said as she stood, and added, "Come on, Horace, let's leave the artists to their work." She grabbed the bag of lichee nuts and headed for the door. She turned on her heel and said, "I hope you're successful—I hope you become the next Jasper Johns!" And she stormed down the stairs.

Soon after, Diego had invited us to Indochine, Brian McNally's popular French-Vietnamese restaurant that had just opened on Lafayette Street, with its palm-frond wallpaper like that of the Beverly Hills Hotel. While we were being seated, a couple beckoned Diego over. He returned to tell us we were joining them. Julian Schnabel introduced himself and his wife, Jacqueline.

Starting with his first show at Mary Boone in 1979, Julian Schnabel became a very famous artist. Many people considered him an enfant terrible. He quickly rose to fame in his twenties, gluing broken plates, saucers, and cups to boards and topping them with bold paint strokes; painting on black velvet; or gluing animal skins and antlers onto paintings. He later told me Holly Solomon had offered to represent him in the seventies but he had opted for Mary Boone.

Julian had a big personality and enormous charm; he was generous, too, and could draw you into his world with his outspoken and entertaining viewpoints. At Indochine he ordered the whole menu. At least it seemed like he did to us. He looked at the menu and spoke to the waitress. "You like shrimp?" he asked us. We nodded. "Okay, let's have two—no, three—shrimp plates. Oh, you've got to try the noodles. We'll have three noodles and three spring rolls—no, four." In minutes the table was covered with plates piled high with food and cold champagne. We were thrilled and ate all of it. Jacqueline was a tall, thin beauty decked out in glamorous attire, with her auburn curls just hitting her shoulders and a huge yellow diamond on her finger. But the best thing about her was her kind personality. I usually found beautiful women intimidating and cold, especially one with a famous and powerful man by her side. Jacqueline was the exact opposite. She was relaxed, funny, and sweet. At the time I didn't realize what an important person she would be in my life. The five of us had a chatty dinner. I was relieved to find out they actually were quite nice, since Julian had such a reputation for being bossy and domineering.

During the lively meal David got up from the table. After a long while Julian asked where my friend was. I excused myself and went to look for him. I found him lying in a small back sitting room (it was really a hallway), splayed out on a bamboo lounge chair and holding his jaw.

"What are you doing?" I asked.

"Oh, my tooth hurts," he whispered in pain.

"Since when?"

"I don't know. When I sat down." He was always having tooth problems.

"Sir, you can't sleep here," called a waiter.

"Come on," I said. "Get up. Everyone's asking for you. And you're missing all the food." I helped him up out of the chair.

"Hey, man, where were you?" Julian asked as we arrived back at the booth.

"Oh, I have a toothache."

"You better get to the dentist," Julian suggested. David nodded, holding his jaw, and picked at the remains of the plates. Then the table was filled with desserts.

On our way back home, his toothache went away. "I guess I was nervous meeting him." McD had a thing about powerful people. Only a few, such as Julian, escaped his untimely, ferocious rages.

About a week later we were walking uptown on Park Avenue (probably going to get money from Vivian) and a voice called out from a cab. It was Julian and Jacqueline, who stopped the cab to say hello. "We're off to India—we'll call you when we return."

At this time we were going back and forth between Catskill and the city where we were still living in the Bowery with Kristian and Bradley. Kristian had been under constant attack from Bradley whose drug addiction had become more apparent. One day Kristian came running into our room with blood streaming down his face, crying that Bradley had thrown a large glass beer stein at him. "I can't stand it any longer here. I'm moving back to California. Please don't tell anyone—especially Bradley."

His plan was to move during the night while Bradley was working at Beulah Land, a bar on Avenue A. That would leave us at the mercy of Bradley, whose behavior was only getting worse. I couldn't believe Kristian would be able to move his belongings in one evening. He had two huge showcases filled with Donny and Marie dolls, Kiss action figures, and endless Beatles memorabilia. We decided to visit friends in Hudson that weekend, and bade Kristian goodbye and good luck.

When we returned Sunday night, Bradley met us at the door in a rage. "What the hell is going on here?" he screamed at us. We pretended to be surprised as he showed us the empty showcases.

Soon Bradley's heroin intake escalated. "I want you out at the first of the month!" he informed us harshly one day. David told him that was

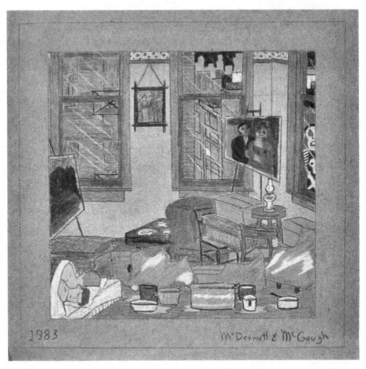

We slept on the floor at McD's Bowery studio with the pots and pans to catch the leaks. Bradley is harassing us through the window.

not going to happen. One night after we had gone to bed we heard his voice chanting in our room, "Get—out—get—out—get—out—of—my—house!" I turned on the light and saw his head was popping out of a gap in the wall under the sink. He stuck his tongue out at me and, like a rabbit, his head went back into the hole. Whenever we were out, he would go into our room and take money and little antiques we had. One night I confronted him as he sat there with a vase and a crucifix he had taken from us sitting on his coffee table. "I don't know what you're talking about," he said, looking right at me.

Then there were the firecrackers he'd throw out his window into ours. One night we came home to find a pile of garbage heaped in front of our door so dense we could hardly open it. David went downstairs and called the police from a pay phone. When they came down the old hallway filled with rubbish and boxes, Bradley jumped out of his doorway in capri pants with a purple fright wig and a large pink plastic caveman club, screaming. He scared us all; one cop punched him, and Bradley fell back into his apartment. The police looked over the pile of garbage and our room with half the ceiling missing and a single bed and asked, "Can't you find a better place to live?" Afterwards, they went in and spoke to a screaming Bradley, and David turned to me and said, "I think it's time to move."

We didn't want to pay the new East Village rents, which could be as much as eight hundred dollars for four rooms. Through an artist/critic Nicolas Moufarrege, Chuck's new boyfriend, we took the top floor above him in an old townhouse on Avenue C and Seventh Street. Again, Vivian came to the rescue and gave us the funds. Immediately McD went into his "de-vinylization" phase, stripping the modern kitchen with the persistence of one possessed and putting it out on the curb, where it disappeared almost immediately. We bought a new metal trashcan and put it outside. That was gone in an hour. He then took out the electricity and covered the electric box up and plastered over it. We painted the rooms dark colors and set up house with antiques from the street or what we could buy for pennies.

When the landlord came over, he was livid at what we had done to his apartment, so I made sketches of what we planned to do to the place and, oddly, he accepted our ideas. David left the bathroom alone, since the claw tub (the exterior of which we painted terra-cotta to look like a clay pot) and the pull-chain toilet from the 1900s were still there, but he tore out the new sink. "You can wash your hands in the bathtub," he said.

He then tore out the three new radiators: "You can sit by the fire if you're cold." He bought lumber, found a blue police barrier, and built two mantels for the front and back working fireplaces. We had them marbleized and we painted a Hudson River School–like painting on the one in the back bedroom and built wooden window frames. David's skills were plentiful.

Diego's representing us did not last and we were soon on our own again. Whenever we were walking home, we'd walk back through Alphabet City only on East Seventh Street between B and C, where drugs were sold, because it was crowded, and the streetlights worked, while the other streets were deserted and dark. The dealers ruled the

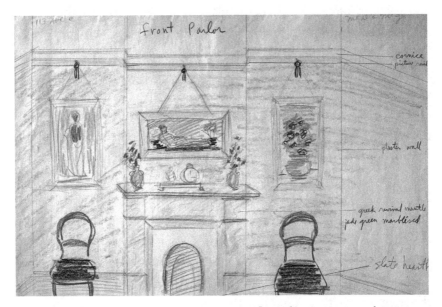

My drawing of our plans for the Avenue C top floor, done to appease the landlord after David's "de-vinylization"

block. From a businessman in suit and tie holding a leather briefcase to a strung-out punk, people were in a line outside an empty, windowless building, being yelled at if they complained or moved out of line. More than a few times it included people we knew. We'd be polite and ignore that we spotted them. Every day, all day long: a bucket with a rope went up with the money and came down with the drugs. Since that was our safe walking block, the drug dealers knew us by sight in our summer linen suits or winter black capes and top hats. One night when we were walking home, a dealer shouted to a junkie who was harassing us. He called from across the street, "Hey! You leave those two alone!" I guess we were the street mascots.

Outside our house was an ice-cream truck, even in January. I couldn't understand why people wanted ice cream when it was so cold out, but it all became clear when one day the police busted the drug ring that used it. And there were many times when we'd hear guns going off during the night. Not many friends wanted to visit us. They couldn't believe we lived so far east in such a neighborhood. If Rome was known as the City of Cats, the East Village was the City of Rats. On our corner I saw a cop who had caught a huge rat in an upside-down plastic milk-carton holder and was stabbing it to death with a broken broomstick.

Many buildings were completely burnt out or just a pile of rubble. Some squatters took over a few and set up house in them. Others were crack dens used for taking drugs. Tenth Street between Avenues C and D was a whole block that was just flat dirt. Then a movie company came and built a tenement to look like the ones we knew so well. We'd take the few who dared to visit in the daytime over to see the set. Of course, there was police protection. The movie was called *batteries not included* (1987), about old people being forced out of their apartments and then saved by tiny spaceships.

Speaking of movies, at the time filmmakers liked to show that starving artists lived in big lofts with beautiful furniture. That was not the case. Just look at Nan Goldin's photographs, which captured the downtown scene of sex, drugs, art, and the disarray of beautiful, messy slumlike interiors. And later her images of friends suffering or dying of AIDS. I recently saw her famous slide show at MoMA and recognized most people in the photos. Although I didn't know Nan well then, our worlds overlapped through a similar circle of friends. It seemed that most everyone we knew in the art world or the punk scene was on heroin. McD used to tell me, "I thought I had to do drugs because the cool people did drugs. But I didn't want drugs. I wanted a black-and-white ice-cream soda."

When Massimo Audiello was building his gallery on East Eleventh Street in 1984, his contractor's boyfriend was ill and dying. It was difficult for Massimo, because he needed his gallery to open on time and yet he was aware of the seriousness of the illness. It's almost impossible to convey to a young person today what it was like then, when so little was known about AIDS.

We went to see our downstairs neighbor and friend the artist Nicolas Moufarrege in the hospital. Chuck was there. All the nurses were in full scrubs with gloves and masks. Chuck, McD, and I were the few not in them. There was a plastic bottle hooked to his bed, so he could urinate. I took the very full bottle after Nicolas asked me to empty it and poured it into the toilet. After I did, the nurse reprimanded me. She was hostile to Nicolas and wasn't very friendly to his visitors. Nicolas died at age thirty-six in 1985. As so often happened, everything was thrown out of his apartment. David went through the belongings and took all the colored threads that Nicholas used for his art to mend our clothes.

In 1987 Oprah Winfrey had a show about a man who had AIDS and swam in a public pool. She went to Virginia to speak to the town. All hell broke loose in the audience, and the people there were livid about the man and his disease. It pretty much summed up the times. Homophobia reared its ugly head, and people all over were concerned. I remember hearing another AIDS casualty, Gordon Stevenson from the no-wave band Teenage Jesus and the Jerks, declare, "Mosquitoes will pass on the disease." No one knew how it was transmitted till later. Aside from hospital visitors having to wear masks and gloves to

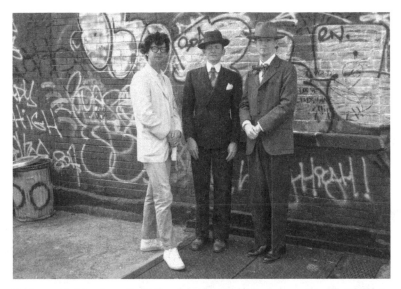

Posing with Massimo Audiello, our second art dealer, outside his Eleventh Street gallery, 1985

visit someone with AIDS, at meals in restaurants and at dinner parties people paused in fear to see which plate or fork or glass was theirs. There was so much shame for the ones who had AIDS, and they were so noticeable in their appearance, with shrunken faces or Kaposi's sarcoma sores. From the pulpit gays were scorned, too. These were men who were shamed for being gay since childhood and then as adults contracted AIDS. The writer Larry Kramer was warning gay men to stop having sex and to close the bathhouses. Some of them were angry and thought they were being put down. They were part of the sexual revolution and didn't want to be told what to do. William F. Buckley, the conservative writer, suggested all AIDS patients be tattooed with a marking to warn others. Many conspiracy theories were floating around about germ warfare, as well as direct condemnation: that blacks and gays—or "niggers and faggots," as they put it—didn't matter; they deserved what they got. I remember a poster that was plastered all over downtown: a red, black, and white image promoting the germ-warfare theory. I heard the man who designed it disappeared.

McD didn't believe in AIDS: "It's erroneous error," he would say, and quote Christian Science founder Mary Baker Eddy, who proclaimed the unreality of "sin, sickness, [and] death." McD, because of his convictions, felt at ease with our sick friends, bringing them healthy vegetarian meals and fresh juices from Angelica's Kitchen on East Twelfth, our favorite restaurant then. He tended to them by changing their dirty bedding, washing them, and putting oils on their sores. Some were shocked by his kindness because they told him most of their friends wouldn't see them. Our friend Simon Bowden, an antiques dealer who lived with us for about six months in 1986 on Avenue C, became ill and moved back to England. When David was visiting London, he hid Simon in his hotel room and took care of him for a week, keeping the Do Not Disturb sign on the doorknob. Simon was shocked that David would share his bed and care for him. McD told me he last saw Simon when they left the hotel and were sitting in a park. Simon lamented this would be the final time he saw David. "Of course we'll see each other again!" David consoled him. Simon died soon afterward. Nobody really knew where this epidemic was going. Out of fear I put my head in the sand. I couldn't bear it. I went along with McD's Christian Science dogma of "no sin, sickness, or death." In fact I was truly terrified.

At Danceteria, in 1979, I had worked with Haoui Montaug, a funny-looking sweetheart who was a doorman at the clubs. He had his own performance evening there called "No Entiendes"—You Don't Understand. It was where Madonna performed. Haoui came down with the famous "cold" that everyone feared. The onset of AIDS usually felt like getting a bad flu. When it didn't go away, a person reluctantly went to get tested. Haoui tested positive. Like all of us, Haoui had seen the horrible devastation of our friends who had suffered a long, harsh illness and a painful death. We all heard he decided to take his own life at a party. In 1991 he invited his closest friends and held a banquet and then took a handful of pills while people said their goodbyes. I was told Madonna was on the phone with him. In 1986 she had lost her best friend and manager Martin Burgoyne who was just twenty-three, a curly-headed blond beauty, and later, Keith Haring, among many others. Ethyl Eichelberger, a drag queen who played the accordion at the

Pyramid Club, took his own life, too, in 1990. How could you blame them? There was no cure or medication that worked—just the horror of impending doom. But Haoui didn't take enough pills and woke up the next morning dismayed. He took twenty more and died in a half hour.

Every week there were funerals and memorials. You'd hear that people you hadn't seen for a while had died. Some went quickly while others lingered in pain with a horrific end. Some had the usual look of swollen bellies and shrunken faces or, like me, had the spots of Kaposi's sarcoma: large purple welts all over their skin that resembled swollen bruises. There was a huge amount of shame around AIDS. Infected people didn't want others to know because they could lose their jobs or be ostracized; there was also the shame of feeling that they had done something wrong or were being punished for having a certain lifestyle. Warhol's somewhat boyfriend Jon Gould was vice president of corporate communications at Paramount, and Andy asked us to meet with Jon and give him all our movie ideas. We sat in Rumpelmayer's on Central Park South and told him our ideas of people in the past coming to the present or people in the present going to the past. Jon became sick, like many others, was down to 70 pounds, blind, and died in 1986. I heard gossip that Andy had freaked out and didn't want to touch Jon's things.

We never got tested. I didn't want that death sentence hanging over me. Cookie Mueller recommended a doctor in the West Village. They were taking my blood for a checkup when I heard the doctor whisper to the nurse, "You better use latex gloves with this one," as he was preparing a needle. When they asked me if I wanted an AIDS test, I said no, not wanting to know. I felt healthy enough. But my fear was real.

We went with our friend Jane Webb, who would throw us a sock full of coins out her window on Mulberry Street when we went looking for a meal, to see a healer, Louise Hay, author of *You Can Heal Your Life,* lecturing at a church in the West Village. Hay's book was a metaphysical one that stated most illness was psychosomatic and came from wrong thinking. The church was packed with people looking for an answer. There we saw some very crushing evidence of AIDS: people's thin, fragile faces dwarfed by a baseball cap or a beard they grew to look not so noticeably unwell. Hay passed around a gold fabric heart with puffy wings and asked us to hold it to our hearts and send blessings. It looked like some kind of odd child's toy, but I tried to go along with it. People were trying different types of healing, like macrobiotic food, rather than AZT, which ravaged the body. In 1986 AZT was one of the only drugs they thought worked, but it was very harsh on the system and caused great harm. Those people didn't survive, either.

10

I n 1985, the year FUN closed, a gallery opened on Bleecker and Crosby that, for six months, became the hottest, coolest gallery downtown. The gallery asked to meet with us to make a show for their pumpkin-colored walls. Rene Ricard was there most days, along with Terry Toye, the trans model who worked with Stephen Sprouse and walked Chanel's catwalk in Paris. The gallerist also slept there on the floor. Hip, cute boys hung out wearing eyeliner and black leather jackets. Warhol and Mary Boone showed up at one opening. Maripol opened a fashion boutique across the street, and Madonna (Maripol styled her famous look) let her use her name for a line of jewelry with multiple plastic rubber hoop earrings and bracelets. And then Madonna changed her style to a blond Marilyn Monroe look.

David came up with the idea of making a ten-foot-wide painting of the crucifixion with Matt Dillon as Christ, singer Billy Idol as a slave, and Attila (the hot male model of the moment) as the good thief. McD made a deal for thirty thousand dollars for the idea. Diego couldn't believe that he did it and giggled when we handed him ten thousand dollars as his cut. We ordered the enormous stretcher and had a cross built and put it in our studio at the Middle Collegiate Church. The gallery had two silent partners. One backer was the brother of a famous fashion photographer who would later die of AIDS and the other was the son of a well-known clothing designer who went to prison. With this money we were going to start the Calvary painting and set ourselves up in the Hudson River Valley to make thirteen paintings depicting Christ and his apostles naked in the landscapes for a show in Naples, Italy, with the famous dealer Lucio Amelio. In only one month we had spent all the money and needed more. Diego yelled at us and said we should have used the money to live on for the next three months.

We found a floor in the Masonic Lodge in Catskill, across from the jail, for our studio. We went to thirteen sites and made sketches. It was somewhat performance-based but was unrecorded except for a photo of me by Vivian at the Delaware Water Gap. McD went immediately into wallpapering mode on the arts-and-crafts Masonic interior with dollar-a-roll paper from an old paint store in Albany. When we were in

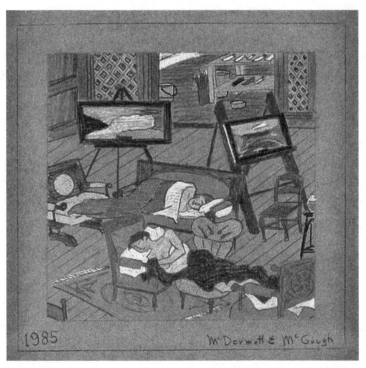

For months, we slept on makeshift beds in our studio in the Masonic Lodge in Catskill.

Albany we'd always stop in a dockworkers' restaurant for the most deli-cious fresh fish sandwich and fries for a dollar fifty. We sat there in high starched collars and high button shoes among the macho truck drivers and dockworkers smoking at the counter downing their steins of beer.

Back at the studio McD kept wallpapering. We'd get into arguments when I wanted him to get back to work and help with the paintings. He would shout back, "You're the one who wanted to be an artist! If you wanted to be a hairdresser, we'd have a salon and do marcel waves!" So I would block out the paintings and fill them in, and later David would sit for hours each day painting in tiny leaves, branches, and rocks. Painting with him was easy and enjoyable. On the Bowery I had started a painting of lovers ready to jump over a cliff and then went to see my mother in Syracuse. When I returned, David had blocked out a vista of the Hudson River below them with a steamship. He asked if I liked it. "I love it!" I exclaimed.

For the Hudson River School paintings we took an old tin painting box we had and filled it with new paints, brushes, and glass bottles of linseed oil and turpentine, and then set out with little stretched can-vases to paint at the thirteen chosen sites including Kaaterskill Falls, Catskill Creek, and even Niagara Falls. We left our hotel just near the cascades at sunrise to paint Niagara. But after a few hours, bus after bus of tourists used us as their background for travel pictures and kept asking questions. Not feeling very friendly, and wanting to finish before the place became mobbed, I dashed through the sketch and hurried off. On the bus back to the train we met a beautiful blond fellow who struck up a conversation with us. He knelt on the seat in front of us to chat. We were thrilled that this beauty took an interest in us, and McD was quite enamored and spouted frivolity. Then the blond Adonis asked us, "Do you accept Jesus Christ as your own personal Savior?" David paused and replied, "Well, I think of myself *as* Jesus!" The flaxen god turned silent and sat back down in his seat.

A week later we went into the Adirondacks to paint another vista. After a few hours the sun was setting, so we gathered our belongings and started down the mountain, but we quickly realized we were lost.

We climbed another mountain, and when we arrived at its peak, all we could see was more mountains. I could feel my heart in my throat as the gloaming was upon us. My body was tingling with fear. I remembered from when I was a child my father volunteering to look for a little girl who was lost in this same vicinity for weeks. I didn't say a word, but my mind raced with scenarios of being eaten by bears or coyotes, or two skeletons in Victorian clothes found in the distant future. McD started to sing an old hymn, "He Leadeth Me," as we descended the mountain. I was too scared to get annoyed. Finally, after two hours of searching we came to a farmer's house in a cornfield and found the road back.

We continued to make the thirteen oil sketches to work from for our show in Naples. We brought the sketches back to our studio in the Masonic Lodge in Catskill, but the paintings took longer than we had thought, since David continued wallpapering the arts-and-crafts interior in period papers. We also rented a small apartment in a run-down eighteenth-century house in Athens, New York, which had a barbershop across the street that looked like it could have been the cover of *The Saturday Evening Post.*

We heard that Rene Ricard had bought some thrift-store paintings and signed them McDermott & McGough & Cortez, and the pumpkin-colored gallery on Bleecker Street that we were making the Crucifixion painting for had a showing of Rene's paintings. We were furious with the gallery, as was Diego, for mocking us so publicly by having this show of fake McDermott & McGough paintings.

We ran into Massimo and he took us for some ice cream and told us he was opening a gallery on East Eleventh Street and Avenue A. In his thick Italian accent, he said, "If you're not working with Diego, I'd like to have you represented in my gallery. It has to be between just us." We let him know we were on our own. He asked us to prepare a show for the gallery. The downstairs parlor-floor apartment on Avenue C became available. Of course, David had to have it. We convinced the landlord that we would use it on a month-to-month agreement, with no lease. We started working furiously on the show. I had to ask McD to stop his "de-vinylization" of the new floor and get to work on the paintings. Other than the Crucifixion, we usually painted small canvases, and McD wanted to make larger paintings. Maybe Schnabel's large canvases had inspired him. When we were in the middle of painting for the future exhibition, Massimo received a lawyer's letter from the Bleecker Street gallery demanding the thirty thousand back or they would stop us from showing with Massimo. Massimo got hysterical. "Where am I going to get thirty thousand dollars?" he cried, as he hung his head in his hands.

There was a pretty young blond southern woman named Candy Coleman who worked at the front desk. She had the sweetest demeanor and McD adored her southernisms. Massimo had mixed feelings. "I don't know what to think of her," he lamented.

"Why?" we asked.

"I don't know. She's nice, but she's . . . ah . . . *too* nice," he continued. "She always seems to be in a good mood: 'Good morning, Massimo. How are you today, Massimo? Can I get you something, Massimo?' Nobody can be this nice or friendly. I think she's hiding something." We burst into laughter.

"She's southern, Massimo," David told him. "It's a southern tradition to be polite."

"Well, I don't know any southerners," he said, thinking it over.

One day he was fretting to Candy about how to get the money. "I have money if you need it," Candy told him.

"Whaaaaaaat!?" Massimo screamed.

Candy set up a contract, and in it she took our best painting, *The Scapegoat*, as part of the deal. The other gallery was paid, and the show went on.

John Patrick Fleming had a beautiful brother, Brian, who looked like a young Joe Dallesandro, the Warhol actor. Brian had been in and out of reform schools and had a muscular prison body with a few homemade tattoos. I started an affair with him. Brian and a young French dancer McD had a crush on would model for us. We made paintings of the two as young lovers full of longing and lost love. I think we made the show in a few months. I'd pose the models and paint in the backgrounds afterwards. McD was good at the details. As we got closer to the opening, we painted full days, and since we didn't use electric light every moment counted. A week before the show opened in 1985, we moved the wet paintings to Massimo's gallery and did the finishing touches there. We had an announcement card printed that read in bold type: ATTENTION AND ATTENTION! COME SEE THE LARGE PAINTINGS OF MCDERMOTT & MCGOUGH. We painted the white gallery two shades of green like the halls of an old school. McD had Massimo buy two large terra-cotta-potted palms and placed them on Persian carpets to hide the cement flooring. We had Brian tend the bar in a vintage white soda-jerk outfit he had worn for a painting that was in the show, one of nine about the life of a young man in the nineteenth century. At the opening, Julian came with Diane Keaton and went about helping to sell the show after he had picked the painting he wanted first. Philip Niarchos bought one, and another collector said, "I'm rich enough to buy one later, to wait and see if they make it." That night the show sold out, with a mob filling the gallery and pouring out into the street. It was a packed house of East Village artists and admirers. Andy came with designer Stephen Sprouse. David took Andy around the show, and he bought a painting of our homoerotic version of Pygmalion. "Can I get an artist discount?" he asked.

David brought Andy over to meet Brian. "Doesn't he look like Joe Dallesandro, Andy?"

"Yeah. Sure. I guess," Andy replied.

McDermott then took Warhol to a corner and told him how we made smaller penis portraits that we weren't showing. He said they were in the back of the gallery, where we showed them privately.

"Oh. I want to see them!" Andy begged.

"Not now, Andy—Massimo put them away. I'll ask him to show you at the end of the opening." I couldn't believe McD was making this all up. As Andy was leaving, he came up to us and asked when he could see the penis portraits. I didn't know how David was going to end this gag. Massimo came up to us and Andy asked about the paintings.

"What!" Massimo laughed, and in his broken English said, "Paintings of-a cocks?" Still laughing, he pulled us away to meet a collector. "Okay, Andy," he said, "we get the cock paintings to-a you."

The crowd thinned out, and we headed to a restaurant in the financial district, an intact old German-style place complete with its entire original wood paneling, crystal chandeliers, and a mural of ancient Egypt. David ordered his favorite meal of a Thanksgiving turkey feast served with all the trimmings, at a long table for eighty people.

The art world was smaller then, and most of the people in it knew one another. SoHo became the Saturday place for going around to the galleries, and Sunday was for the East Village galleries. SoHo galleries were big and dramatic. East Village galleries looked dingy, and Massimo was criticized because his gallery looked more SoHo than East Village, with high ceilings, perfect white walls, and a polished cement floor. He was also criticized for being friends with such successful SoHo artists as Francesco Clemente and Julian Schnabel and their glamorous wives, Alba and Jacqueline.

One Sunday while we were at the gallery to look at the exhibition, David Hockney and Henry Geldzahler walked in. I don't know what the others there thought, but I was dumbstruck. Hockney had been an important influence in my early life. I loved his portraits of Ossie Clark, the English designer, and the one of Geldzahler on his pink sofa. But we left them alone as they looked over the show. I heard later that Hockney thought one of us painted the people and the other did the background. We never had those kinds of rules. We knew each other so well, and the one thing we never fought about was what the other painted.

By the late 1970s, Andy Warhol's contemporaries had lost interest in him and his artwork. They thought he had sold out, hanging with Halston and Liza at Studio 54. And when he appeared on the television show *The Love Boat,* they lost all respect. But my generation loved him.

We all wanted to meet him. Douglas Cramer, an art collector and the producer of *The Love Boat,* told me that Andy said he'd be on the show if Doug could encourage movie stars to have their portraits done. So Doug had a big party with Andy and many famous actors. Andy was in heaven. But the portraits didn't come through, so Cramer commissioned some on his own.

At that time, the art world was more conservative and didn't like the commercial world. They also did not like that Keith Haring had his Pop Shop. Andy took all of that in and he proved to be a big influence and visionary, and now it seems he was way ahead of his time, but his generation felt disdain for him.

The first time I found out how much his generation didn't respect his work was when the art critic Robert Rosenblum and his wife, the artist Jane Kaplowitz, bought a large Warhol self-portrait in red with a shock of hair that went to the top of the painting. They bought it in 1986 from the Anthony d'Offay Gallery in London. Jane told me they had the pick of any painting. The Rosenblums always gathered an interesting group around them—everyone from Jasper Johns, who rarely said much, to Philip Johnson and David Whitney, who were a lot of fun, and other art dealers, critics, and artists. The painting they bought was the only painting that sold in that show at the time. After they installed it in their living room, they were criticized for buying a Warhol. "Why would you want a Warhol?" friends would ask. Robert in his brilliance defended the portrait. There was also a story that at an art fair, when a gallery installed a whole booth of Warhol's work, the galleries on either side complained that their booths, artists, and artwork would suffer because of it. That's how badly his work was regarded. When the art dealer Howard Read wanted to show some of his photographs that he'd sewn together in groups, Andy's main dealer, Leo Castelli, had little interest and said to go right ahead. I once asked Andy if he had seen the latest issue of *Artforum*: his painting of Life Savers was on the cover. "What did they say? I'm too commercial?"

One of the great things about Andy was that we could drop by the Factory on Thirty-Third Street whenever we wanted. Brigid Berlin would usually be at the front desk, doing needlepoint and casting a jaundiced eye on everyone. She knew how to make you uncomfortable, we were extra polite, but it made no difference. David always went up to her: "Good afternoon, Messrs. McDermott and McGough are here to see Andy Warhol." Without a word, she'd pick up the phone. "Those old-fashioned people are here again," she would say, hang up, and go back to her needlepoint.

Andy would appear on a balcony above a taxidermied elephant painted over by Keith Haring. "Oh, hi. Come on up."

At a long table there would be a lunch either starting or ending. We always hoped it was starting. It would be for a celebrity, a client, or advertisers for the magazine. His assistant Ben Liu (drag name Ming Vase) and Paige Powell, his pretty gal Friday, would usually be there. If we had a cute young fellow we were interested in, we would bring him to Andy for the "Wow" effect.

I always felt Andy was clever to surround himself with young people. We all adored him, worshiped him, and wanted to know him.

11

One day David saw a 1930s convertible coupe for sale in the paper. Calling from Massimo's gallery phone (that was where we made calls and received messages, since we didn't have a phone of our own because of both the expense and McD's nineteenth-century aesthetic), he made an appointment with the seller on Long Island. A day or two later we were on the train.

"Where are we going to get the money to buy it, David?"

"Oh, will you please stop! It's only a few thousand, and we can put a deposit down."

"That's for the rent!"

"We can pay that later. Why are you always causing problems, Peter? You're so depressing! We need this for our image and to enrich our lives. Can't you imagine how great it will be driving around in this car?"

"We don't know how to drive!" I yelled.

"We'll get a chauffeur, then!" he barked.

We bickered till the train conductor announced our stop. A man was standing by the described advertised car. I must admit it looked great. It was a dream of an automobile. The owner looked a bit like Porky Pig, round and cute, wearing pastel colors matching the tan convertible coupe. After the introduction he asked who wanted to drive. We looked at each other. "Why don't you show us how it drives first?" David suggested, and winked at me.

"Well, you boys look like the right fit for this car. Where'd you get the getups?"

"We live in the past and that's why we need an old car."

"You live in the past? That's rich," snorted Porky.

I sat in the back, with David up front endlessly chatting to the man about his theories of time travel, his plan for entering another dimension, and how we were definitely buying the car. I could tell the man thought he had a fast sale on his hands, with David bragging how rich and famous he was.

"Where shall we drive? Any place in particular? Don't you boys want to give it a spin?"

With a burst David exclaimed, "Hey, I got a great idea! Why don't we visit our friend Julian Schnabel in Bridgehampton? He just got back from India. He's a really famous artist!"

"Okay, buddy, then we got to backtrack," Porky said as he made a U-turn.

I was a bit nervous about dropping in on Julian. We didn't really know him except for that Indochine dinner and a few chance meetings. Diego had taken us to visit them in Bridgehampton once before. David had an uncanny sense of direction and we managed to find the house. David ran in and came out with Julian and showed him the car. Julian invited us in, but not Porky. I never saw anyone so politely and professionally exclude someone as Julian did. I kind of felt sorry for our driver but was happy he wasn't coming in, too.

"Hey, what about the check?" he yelled as we went inside.

"Oh, we'll mail it later—bye!" waved David. We never bought the car.

The house in Bridgehampton was a 1920s Sears, Roebuck mail-order product, shingled and two-storied, with a front porch for viewing sunsets. In the back, off the kitchen, they had built a screened extension, and outside was an Italian stone arch through which you could see an Olympic-sized swimming pool with a big sculpture of Julian's at one end. Julian had also made an outdoor, three-walled studio with no roof; the paintings and paint tables were covered in plastic sheets and would sit there rain or shine. He'd take tarps, drag them with a truck through the mud and dirt, and paint on them. He was always looking for different materials to work with, from plates to velvet, boxing-ring tarps to painted theater backdrops.

We accepted the Schnabels' offer to stay with them for a few days, and Julian lent us swimsuits that hung on our thin frames. David called their life "relaxed high-tone," but the kindness and inclusiveness they showed us was a great comfort. I'd stare at Jacqueline as she served dinner and got us to try ethnic foods we weren't accustomed to. I'd look up in awe at that beautiful face, smiling as she handed me a plate of food. I had finally met one of the women I adored from the movies I watched on television as a boy.

Julian spent a lot of time in his outdoor studio, and I watched him and his assistant mixing up colors from huge tubes of oil paint into large Chinese-takeout plastic tubs. David and I both sat for plate-painting portraits. Once, as Julian was getting ready to paint, he turned to me: "Hey, why don't you make a painting and use that canvas?" I looked behind me and saw what to me was a mural-sized stretched canvas. Our paintings were usually no bigger than two feet tall. "Come on—go ahead, man," he encouraged me.

I looked at this large mass of white canvas and at his mixed colors that screamed bright in the noonday sun. Out of a vast pile of used brushes I picked a few and gathered some of his plastic tubs of mixed colors and set them in front of me. He was on the other side of the studio, working with his back to me. Years before I had seen in a book on the American cubist painter Stuart Davis a picture of his 1921 soda-fountain mural, now destroyed, at the Gar Sparks Nut Shop in Newark, New Jersey, where the artist painted menu words on the wall in abstract letters of different sizes: "IcE cREam, sOdA, oRanGadE," etc. (Gar Sparks was an artist friend of Davis's, and the top salesman at the 1913 Armory Show, where he sold Duchamp's *Nude Descending a Staircase*.) I loved the photo I saw of it and wanted to use the idea for a painting sometime. David and I had discussed it, but I didn't know what words to use. "How about Civil War battles?" David suggested. "No, that wouldn't work," I thought. But here at Julian's I thought of all the names I had been called since I was a child. The words flooded over me: "faggot," "fairy," "pansy," "nelly," "queer." This was the moment, and I threw myself into it. All those taunts went swirling down on the canvas with the crushing names in different colors. I went wild laying them down for everyone to see. I walked over to the paint table and took more colors in plastic take-out tubs. I didn't care that my suit was paint-splattered. I reveled in it. I thought of all the boys in school as I painted over their catcalls I knew by heart.

"Hey!" I heard Julian yell. "What are you doing?"

Oh, no, I thought, maybe it's too much with all these gay words. "Well, um . . . why, is it too much?" I shyly asked.

"No, man—you're taking all the mixed colors I just made! Never mind—this is great! Keep going." He smiled. Having seen the small, almost empty tubes we usually worked with when he visited our studio, at the end of those days in Long Island he started piling up his large tubes of colors for us, placing them in a bag.

"You'll need cerulean blue, titanium white—of course, maybe two. Then here's some Naples yellow and cadmium red . . . burnt umber," and on and on. We left with a heavy bag of paint.

When we first had Julian and Jacqueline over to Avenue C, he looked at our single mattress and asked why we didn't get a larger one but complimented us on how we'd set up house. His world was so big: with a big studio, big paintings, and a large appetite for life. He'd see an arrangement of figurines on our table and say, "Why not make a painting of this? This is beautiful." He'd often talk with us about his own work or others' paintings, pointing out how colors react to one another. In fact, looking at paintings with him was an art course in itself. He became our mentor, someone we could go to and ask for advice, often about money or art dealers. I saw him help out many artists and some actors, giving or lending them money. Jacqueline was always beyond generous, too.

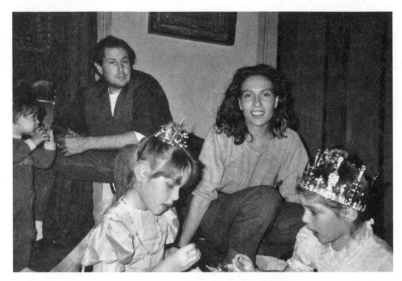

Jacqueline and Julian with Vito, Lola, and Stella, visiting Avenue C for our annual Halloween party for the Schnabel children

Perhaps like most artists I was a mixture of absolute narcissism and crippling self-doubt, but I was eager to learn. I watched him as he painted and as he showed his work to other people. Maria Callas or Iggy Pop would be playing loudly on the stereo. He'd ask his two assistants to move the large paintings around, one after another, then he'd go over each one and speak about the colors, lines, and placement.

We became very close to Julian and Jacqueline, traveling with them and having dinners at their home with their children and friends. Julian introduced us to his European dealers and we started to show with them. He spoke to us about our art and brought great insight to us. He seemed to barge through life, taking control. If we were broke, he'd lend us money, always first asking who owed us from painting sales. Julian lent us his large studio on White Street over the former Mudd Club, a floor-through loft with a double-height ceiling in the front. The Schnabels were using it as a storage space for all the mid-century furniture they collected. The artist Ross Bleckner, who had a studio and living space on the upper two floors, owned the building. We had hired "French Chris," whom McD knew from the downtown scene, to help us. Our Italian dealer, Lucio Amelio, came by and couldn't believe we had such a gorgeous man cleaning up the brushes. Even Massimo went after him. Chris was in a famous photo by Nan Goldin posed passed out on the back of a sixties convertible, and her friend the photographer David Armstrong did many adoring pictures of him. When Ross saw him, he immediately offered him a job. Chris said he could work for us both. David said not to bother and dismissed him. A few weeks later Chris showed up asking for his job back: "It didn't work out upstairs." But we had already hired someone else.

Anyway, it was incredible to have such a large space to work in, so we made larger paintings. Julian had our painting with "cocksucker" and many other words written on it delivered from Bridgehampton. I painted the background yellow and made the word "Mary" in bold red letters.

12

I n 1985 Massimo had the silly but brilliant idea for a group show about Pat Hearn's Chihuahua, Chi-Chi. I first saw Pat when she was singing in a nightclub with McD. She had a beehive hairdo and a long, sixties-style lime-green dress with a large circle cut out below the neckline. She had penciled-in eyebrows that shot up to her hairline and had a gap between her teeth. She reminded me of a spacewoman on the sixties TV show *Star Trek*. Massimo included an early painting of Julian's that had a Chihuahua in it. He asked us as well as Jean-Michel, George Condo, Don Van Vliet (aka Captain Beefheart), and Philip Taaffe, among others. I escorted Massimo to the two-story studio Jean-Michel rented from Warhol on Great Jones Street. The large first floor was the studio, filled with many canvases, paints, and boxes that he had painted on, with an array of work in different stages of completion littering the floor. We climbed a small staircase to an apartment above, decorated with Andy's arts-and-crafts furniture. The beautifully appointed room was a shamble of clothes, shoes, and numerous shopping bags from pricey stores. On the round dark-wood dining table were numerous half-empty wine bottles and glasses. I glanced at a half-empty bottle of Château Margaux. A large ashtray was filled with cigarette butts and joints. A plastic bag of pot sat next to it.

I had first met Basquiat when he was known as a brilliant young artist only on the Lower East Side, before all the fame set in. One day, McD had rung Glenn O'Brien's doorbell on St. Marks Place. David loved to drop in on people. He had known Glenn since the 1970s when Glenn worked at *Interview* magazine. "Hi, Glenn, it's David McDermott," he announced, and the buzzer rang. Glenn was sitting with a cute young black kid. The front of his head was shaved, and he had a bunch of dreadlocks tied together at the back of it. They were smoking a joint. David started a conversation and then began to sing the song "Crazy Rhythm," from the 1920s:

> *They say that when a high brow meets a low brow*
> *Walking along Broadway*
> *Soon the high brow, he has no brow*
> *Ain't it a shame and you're to blame . . .*
> *Crazy rhythm, I've gone crazy too.*

Jean had him repeat it as he wrote down the lyrics on a piece of paper.

In his apartment on Great Jones Street, Jean greeted Massimo and me wearing only pajama bottoms. He was relaxed and friendly as he lit up a joint. Massimo pulled out some Polaroids he'd taken of Chi-Chi and Jean looked them over and crouched down on the floor among some scattered large pieces of paper that had footprints and words already on them. Massimo got down on the floor with him as Jean started to draw Chi-Chi. I've never forgotten that image of Jean drawing on the floor as Massimo complimented him—"Ah, Jean, that's fantastic!"—while I sat on a dining-room chair watching. We all respected his vast talent from the very start.

After his show at Mary Boone on West Broadway in 1984 and the famous photo of him barefoot on the cover of the *Times Magazine* in 1985, word on the street was that he was over. People started saying he had lost his talent, he was a drug addict, he had AIDS, he was hanging around Warhol too much. Then the collectors started to lose interest, with some dumping his work at auction houses. His last show before his death in 1988 was at Vrej Baghoomian's gallery in the Cable Building at Broadway and Houston; Baghoomian was Tony Shafrazi's cousin, and the invitation had a shadowy photograph of Jean showing how bad his skin looked as he held a copy of Jack Kerouac's *The Subterraneans.* This show was a step down from the larger galleries he was used to. We went to the opening with the rest of the mob from the East Village. It was packed with his friends and admirers.

Jean eventually pulled out of *The Chi-Chi Show,* leaving Massimo upset. He had known Jean from the beginning, through Diego, and he had put Jean's name on the list of the exhibiting artists in a full-page ad in *Artforum.* "Jean says he's not going to be in the show—well, fuck him! We'll still have a great show!" he screamed. I could see how upset Massimo was.

Julian installed the show for Massimo, beautifully arranging each work. One painting he thought was weak he hung near the top of the high ceiling. But we had other plans for our painting *The Scapegoat* and took a small wall in the front of the gallery desk by the large windows. We had worked diligently on our painting: since we were in a group show with such bold-faced names, we knew we had to make the "best in show." We had found a Victorian gold frame in a junk shop and had it restored on the Bowery. Our painting was of a naked young man asleep on our Empire sofa in our blue-colored parlor on Avenue C; he was the dancer from France that David had a crush on. The young man lay prostrate on the sofa in a disheveled room. We painted our favorite Pre-Raphaelite paintings hanging askew on the wall behind him. The door to the room had been left ajar from an overnight guest's departure, and little Chi-Chi (painted from a Polaroid Massimo gave us) was jumping up to wake the boy. We papered the gallery wall with a scrap of pink Victorian wallpaper and with another scrap of wallpaper that had a decorative border in blue. The painting hung from a silk-covered picture wire with a tassel, hooked onto a colored picture rail. We hung it at an angle like the ones in the painting. No spotlight was used, only the natural light from the street.

At the dinner after the opening of *The Chi-Chi Show*, McD stood on a tabletop and sang as he tiptoed through the glassware. McD was famous for singing at art parties and dancing on the tables between the empty plates and glasses, even jumping from one table to another, to the awe of the diners. At Mr Chow in New York he'd slide down the brass banister and take command of the room as he sang, "I am a butterfly and cannot sing, but in a moment the birdies will teach me." He then was asked by other artists to come to their dinners and sing. It made some of the boring ones much more fun.

When International with Monument opened on East Seventh Street in 1984, four emerging artists—Jeff Koons, Ashley Bickerton, Peter Halley, and Meyer Vaisman—got a lot of press, and the collectors thronged to the space. The graffiti movement of all the kids from the Bronx had died out. The fury of snapping up those spray-paint paintings waned; and those kids, who for the first time had had gobs of cash and spent it on cars and clothes, now had to go back to jobs. (An ungenerous reviewer writing in a free uptown magazine noted that graffiti was "the briefest artistic movement on the record; the art world equivalent of the Nehru jacket.") One artist went back to his bike-messenger job. Fab 5 Freddy, né Fred Brathwaite, starred on *Yo! MTV Raps*. Out of that group only Jean-Michel, Keith Haring, and Kenny Scharf moved on and thrived. In 1985 there were almost seventy galleries in the East Village. By 1987 almost all of them closed and a remaining few moved to SoHo. The East Village scene was disappearing. Rents were increasing more than six times over; collectors lost interest in that art, and people were dying or moving elsewhere from the devastation of AIDS. But Massimo managed to continue to sell our work. Pat Hearn had sold her nude portraits by Warhol and built an immense gallery between Avenues C and D. In 1986 we did a double show with Massimo and Pat. Pat was worried that we weren't going to finish her show, which consisted of forty small genre paintings. The paintings we made for Massimo's show were large "time maps." We blocked out abstract colors on large canvases and put dates in the different color blocks. Each painting represented a century. Pat's show sold well, but Massimo's didn't—the paintings were too different from what the collectors and critics were used to from us.

Many artists show every other year or so, but as Massimo's best-selling artists, we showed every year from 1985 to 1988. Unlike some galleries in the East Village, he paid us right away; when he was paid, we were paid. One day Massimo called and asked us to get ready for Richard Marshall, one of the curators of the 1987 Whitney Biennial. I had never met a museum curator before, so in my panic I hid the large yellow painting *A Friend of Dorothy* behind a group of large stretchers Julian had left. I went downstairs and outside to wait for him and anxiously kept looking at the few people who walked by on White Street. A few minutes later, a man in glasses came up to me and introduced himself: "Hi, I'm Richard." We had tea and cookies for him, and I let David walk him through the work in the studio as I stuffed the wafers into my mouth and rearranged the ones left to fill the now almost empty plate.

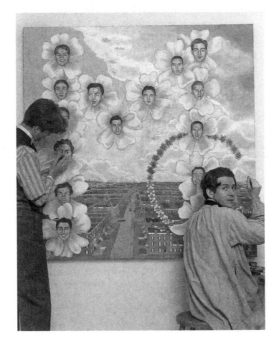

I am on the left as we finish *The Daisy Chain* in Mario Diacono's Boston gallery for our 1987 show.

He didn't say much, but he nodded at David's explanations. As he was leaving, he spotted a long strip of yellow hiding behind the stretchers.

"What's that?" he asked.

"Oh, just something we are working on," I replied nervously.

"May I see it?" he asked.

I was a bit hesitant because no one really had seen the painting yet with its words that seemed so harsh. I pulled the painting out and leaned it against a wall. Richard stared at it in silence. I thought, "Okay, were finished now. We won't get in."

After an endless pause he looked over at us and said, "Why were you hiding this? It's wonderful!" I never expected that reaction, and suddenly all my nervousness was gone. We then became exuberant and started explaining the work. When it was dry, Massimo had it delivered to his gallery. We later went over and found Pat Hearn admiring the new work. Massimo had a great collector hold the painting and a private dealer said it could never be resold because of words like "cocksucker." The client dropped the offer, and Jane and Robert Rosenblum bought it.

Weeks later, Massimo called and told us that we were included in the 1987 Biennial. They chose three paintings to be included. *Rub-a-Dub-Dub . . . Three Boys . . . and One Tub* was a painting we made from a 1930s Bon Ami advertisement of a father and two young boys in a bathroom, but we painted them all naked; *The Time Tunnel,* with David walking into a swirling mass of dates; and the abstract word painting *A Friend of Dorothy,* slang for homosexuals after the character of Dorothy in *The Wizard of Oz.* Since Judy Garland was the gay man's idol, they would go to a party and ask, "Are there any friends of Dorothy here?"

We wore full dress tails to the Whitney opening and stood in front of our painting because Holly Solomon had once told us Warhol always stood in front of his paintings at openings. Two men came up to us and said we had stolen Editta Sherman's walking stick, which David was holding. McD instantly held it out and said, "Here, you can return it." The strangers turned, then walked away, grimacing. Our work was

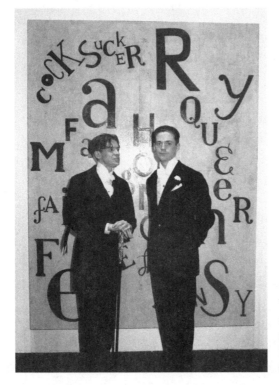

We are in white ties in front of *A Friend of Dorothy* at the 1987 Whitney Biennial; David is holding Editta Sherman's walking stick.

hailed in the press as some of the strongest in the show. Mike and Doug Starn received a lot of attention for their beautiful photo-and-tape images of a dead Christ. And lurking just around the corner from our room was the Jeff Koons fish tank with basketballs. When we brought Vivian to the Biennial and showed her our room, she asked, "With all the words in the English language you had to use those?"

In the early eighties when we were first starting out, we heard through Diego about the Swiss art dealer Bruno Bischofsberger. But nothing happened, though he liked the few paintings Diego showed him. There were many rumors going around about Bruno, such as that he was from a family of rich chocolate merchants, but in fact his father was a dentist. He started selling Swiss primitive art and then went on to contemporary. His daily dress was knee britches, a collarless jacket, and a cape. Through Julian we became friendlier and realized Bruno was no ordinary dealer and was also one of the most discerning collectors. He bought many works from us. He collected not only glass (he had a Mapplethorpe photograph of his collection), but ceramics, photography, modernist furniture, primitive paintings, and much else. But what I really loved was his collection of pine-needle spheres, from large as a softball right down to small as a marble. They're made of pine needles that fall into lakes and are swirled into spheres by the rippling currents that turn them in circles.

We were in the middle of making a show for Massimo in the White Street studio, and we were again desperate for money. When we went to Massimo to ask, he said, "I don't have any money! Don't ask me for any money—not even a penny!" Then, when we were making a new show to open around the time of the Whitney Biennial, Massimo said to us, "Make some paintings that I can sell!" I was a bit peeved at this request, so I went on to make a painting of a still life taken from an old advertisement card with a vase of flowers in front of a windowed winter landscape. I made the flower arrangement into a big dollar sign. I thought, "This will get him if he wants money paintings." We called Julian to ask for a loan which we had done before. He was with Bruno and he said they would come by later that day. Julian and Bruno arrived at the studio and after a friendly greeting Bruno looked over the paintings and asked if he could buy up the whole roomful of new work—ten paintings. We were thrilled and flattered as Bruno was a well-known and respected dealer and no one had ever wanted to buy that much work at one time; he gave us a few thousand dollars in cash.

Then Massimo wanted to visit. I thought perhaps I could make more paintings to appease both parties. But I was dreaming; our paintings took a long time to make. Massimo came to the White Street studio to see how our work was progressing. I had the uncomfortable task of having to tell him Bruno had bought them all. When I did, Massimo threw his glasses across the room and started screaming. I don't think David was there, and I don't remember much else other than that after his ranting he left. Julian called the next day and said Massimo had called him and that Bruno wouldn't keep the paintings, but wanted to hold on to the dollar-sign bouquet. Of course, the show went on, and

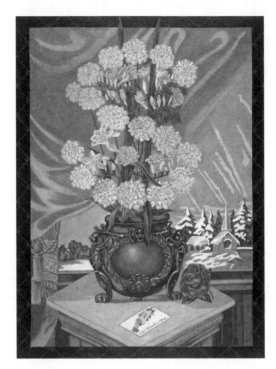

A painting made for
Massimo, who'd asked
for one "that I can sell"

Massimo did sell them all. It was a new world for us having good sums
of money coming in, so that we didn't have to spend most of our day
looking for a meal or hiding from the landlord. But with McD buying
antiques, the money went out as fast as it came in.

Justin Hoag had a shop on East Ninth Street, where he slept in an
old wooden bed behind a curtain. We'd always run into him on our
weekend-morning visits to the flea market in a parking lot on Sixth
Avenue, rain or shine. Justin knew the dealers there and had nicknames
for them all. Twin brothers were "the Twits"; a large, unpleasant woman
was "Fat and Ugly"; a very elderly man was "Sea Hag"; and a heavyset
middle-aged Italian man, dressed in out-of-date seventies clothing, was
"Fat Frank." We found Justin there one Sunday, cackling and carrying
on with Fat Frank. Justin had picked up a Meissen figurine. He had a
knack of getting the best on the tables first. He held it up: "Fraaaaank,
how much?"

"Ten dollars, Justin," Frank said without looking up.

"What? Ten dollars? For this dreck? It has a crack—look," he said, pointing.

"Ten dollars, Justin. I've seen it. It's a hairline fracture."

"Come on, Frank, please . . . I'll give you seven," he flirted and begged. I knew that the figurine was much more valuable even with the crack in it. "Okay, okay—seven, Justin." Justin dug into his paper bag, handing me his now cold cup of coffee. "Please be careful with that," he said.

"It's cold," I said.

"I'm still enjoying it," he snapped with bulging eyes. He rummaged through loose ten-, twenty-, and fifty-dollar bills covering the bottom of his packed paper bag from Henri Bendel on Fifty-Seventh Street ("Rich people shop here," he'd say, pointing to the bag). "Here!" He handed Frank a crumpled five and two dollar bills and dumped his find into the bag.

In front of Cooper Union, between Bowery and Lafayette, people would set up blankets and sell items. Many a time we'd pass by and pick up some old objects. John Patrick would be there sometimes, making some pocket money, shouting, "Good merch—cheap prices!"

13

On Sunday, February 22, 1987, we were in a taxi coming from a Christian Science church service on the Upper West Side when the radio announced that Andy Warhol had died. We immediately told the driver to change directions and to go to Jacqueline and Julian's on Twentieth Street and Broadway. We didn't know where else to go. We rang the buzzer and went upstairs. There were Julian, Jacqueline, and Tony Shafrazi watching the television news of Andy's death. Tony had just had a show of the paintings Andy and Jean-Michel had done together. Only one painting sold, and Julian was the buyer. Pictures of Andy from different periods—with his superstars, at gallery shows—along with his artwork, magazine covers, and everything he influenced were flashing on the screen. On Julian's walls were an *Orange Car Crash,* a *Tunafish Disaster,* and a very large diptych of Julian, all by Andy.

"Did anyone call Paige?" asked Julian. Paige Powell had been Jean-Michel's girlfriend at one time and had worked at *Interview* magazine in the eighties first as an advertising associate and later as associate publisher. We were all so shocked. Andy had been a big part of our lives.

Andy's business partner, Fred Hughes, put a lockdown on the business and brought in Ed Hayes as the lawyer. We went to the funeral at

St. Patrick's on Fifth Avenue. A packed house of boldface names from the Factory, Studio 54, and the art world as well as writers, fashion designers, and more packed the church. John Richardson, the Picasso biographer, and Yoko Ono were two of the speakers.

When we had been in Naples in 1986 for our show with Lucio Amelio we saw that some of the city walls were covered with black-edged paper with pictures of people who had died. McD said this would make a good artwork down the road and went to the printers where they gave us a blank sheet. We produced the Warhol memorial poster and paid for it to be typeset and plastered all over downtown. At an opening at Pat Hearn's new gallery on Ninth Street, we passed out the posters to whoever wanted one.

Through Paige we were invited, with a group, to see Andy's house on East Sixty-Sixth Street. None of the paper bags of loot were visible. Jed Johnson, Andy's former boyfriend, had decorated it in different styles with different periods of furniture, from French modern to Egyptian revival to Early American. Each room was different, and McD and I were fascinated by what was on display. A large bust of Napoleon was

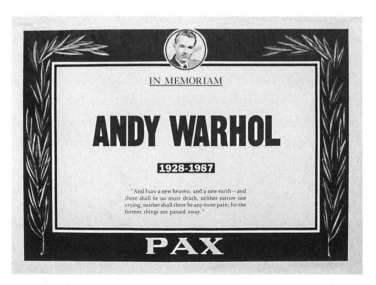

Warhol memorial poster that we made based on memorial posters in Naples. Trey Speegle did the layout after David's design.

on a round Federal table at the entrance. And he had a great collection of modern art. Some wanted it to be kept as a museum, but it all went to auction. Ricky Clifton was there every day and bid on things that didn't go for much and went around town selling them to people he knew.

From Ricky we bought a blanket chest from the 1840s and an eighteenth-century bench we used in the kitchen upstate. There was so much money in the eighties that people were paying a fortune for a cookie jar from the 1930s. One man reportedly paid $198,605 for five lots of them. When Warhol died in 1987, his work was not commanding high prices, but by 1994 that changed—everybody wanted it.

In the beginning of the summer of 1988 Chuck was living in Paris and ran into Jean-Michel on the street. Jean had a huge boil on his forehead and asked Chuck where to score dope. Chuck answered that he didn't do it any longer and didn't know. The next day he walked by a restaurant and saw Jean sitting by the window alone. A few months later he heard Jean was dead.

As a memorial to his friend, Keith Haring painted a pile of crowns honoring the three-pointed crown Jean used in his work. The next year Keith was diagnosed with AIDS. At the time, it was a death sentence, since there was no drug that worked. Keith died in 1990 at age thirty-one. I was at a dinner years later at the Odeon when a modeling agent who was a friend of Keith's remembered him telling her he was upset that what would end up being his last show hadn't sold. These three great friends and artists—Andy, Jean-Michel, and Keith—who were considered yesterday's news before they died, would all once again become best-selling artists, with Andy and Jean-Michel achieving auction records.

In 1987 Diego was curating a show at a well-known prep school in New England—a group show with artwork by Basquiat, McD & McG, and others. At the opening we were surrounded by the faculty and students. One young fellow caught my eye as he came up to me. He was small in stature with green eyes and a mound of brown curls and a disheveled preppy look. He seemed a bit tipsy as he approached. He inquired why one of our paintings, *Lot Leaving Sodom and Gomorrah,* was slashed. I made up something meaningful instead of telling him how McD in a caffeine frenzy had slashed the painting and we had just left it that way. Another art student came up and asked me the same question, and before I knew it a crowd had surrounded me. The wife of the gallery director was trying to pry me away with the promise of some wine. Later I heard her stage-whisper to a teacher, "What a cliché, a bunch of fags from New York!"

As we left, I gave the tousled young man my engraved card (the size of a paperback book) and said, "Call me if you ever need my assistance"—an offer that would evolve into a monumental disaster. I'll name him Sebastian, or Bastian for short. It gives me some emotional distance, making it easier to tell this part of my story.

I later remembered that in 1987 we had made a painting from an old illustration that had three men's faces. It hung in Massimo's gallery, and I had made one of the men a blond youth with blue eyes; at the

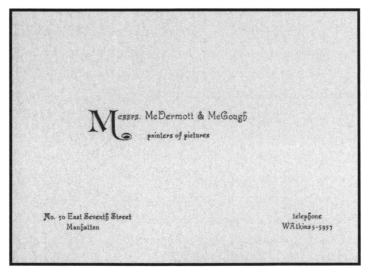

The calling card I gave to Bastian with the church studio address

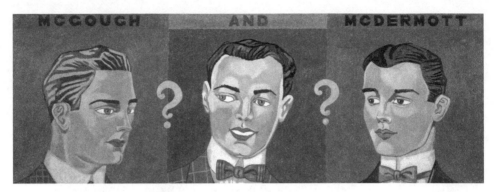

Looking for and . . . 24 x 60, oil on linen, 1921/1987, my painting that somehow foretold the arrival of Bastian.

other end was a redhead with brown eyes; and in the middle I painted an auburn-haired youth with green eyes. Question marks divided the three faces. Had I created a talisman?

A couple of weeks later we did receive a phone call from the young man. He was complaining that his friend had been expelled from the school. McD took the call in our studio on an old wooden crank telephone. I listened in on the extension. David arranged for him to visit us.

The three of us went to the Whitney to see our paintings in the Biennial. It was spring 1987, and Warhol had died in February. Bastian seemed very young and out of his element in the crowd of artists, collectors, and the odd celebrity. He told us he had been given a four-year scholarship to the prep school, talked about his interest in horses (he was a dressage rider), sailing, and his passion for reading. His politics were to the extreme right: he was a fan of the archconservative William F. Buckley. But that didn't faze McD, because he had his dream before him: a beauty with brains. And McD thought he could bring anyone around to his way of thinking. He was a master of conversation when he wanted something, and he had that something right in front of him. His monologues could shock or charm. And he was now hovering with wings of charm in full span. I don't think they ever stopped talking, so I went back to look at the rest of the Biennial. McD would bring up many different subjects as Bastian tried to take them in.

As we were walking back downtown, David said taxis killed conversations and that he preferred to figure out his theories walking. In Bastian's short weekend stay, I could see him and McD interacting with ease. David pulled out all the stops and let Bastian bask in his admiration and compliments. As we took him to the train for his trip back, he paused and asked us to lend him two hundred and fifty dollars—around eight hundred dollars today.

"Of course we can!" McD happily replied.

But it didn't seem right to me. I didn't even know this person, and he was already asking for money. That red flag was flying high, but all I could see was his pretty face.

A few weeks later we received a long thank-you letter saying how much he'd enjoyed the stay, with no mention of the money.

We were planning to rent a place on Capri for the month of August, and we asked Bastian if he would assist us in the studio there, an offer he accepted. We had rented our friend Paola Igliori's house. Paola, a slim beauty with wild hair that hovered around her face, was then married to the artist Sandro Chia; she was a descendant of Pope Julius II, who commissioned Michelangelo to paint the Sistine Chapel. When an Italian dry cleaner asked her if she was related to the kings of Italy, she said, "I'm from a much better family!"

Paola was aristocratic and bohemian with a soft, mellifluous voice. We flew to Rome and took the train to her beautiful estate, Villa Lina, two hours outside the city. The same landscape architect who designed the gardens of Villa Borghese had designed hers. There was a walnut orchard and a waterfall that cascaded through carved shells to a pond below. Mussolini once swam in the large swimming pool which was surrounded by columns of trees with a striped cabana tent at the end. During World War II, the locals broke the gate and went up the drive lined with horse chestnut trees and squatted in the main house. Supposedly the father, on his return, chased them out and tore down the house, leaving only the wine cellar. Paola lived in the servants' quarters, surrounded by the paintings and furniture of her once grand family. We stayed with her a few days before leaving for Capri. One day Cy Twombly came to lunch. He was a tall, charming man in a white linen suit. He had attracted the attention of the art world like his close friends Robert Rauschenberg and Jasper Johns, though some people were still saying they didn't like Twombly's work. The same went for Lucian Freud, and hardly anyone was interested in Francis Bacon. But, in fact, Cy was beloved in the art world. He had great support and many admirers, and continues to influence younger generations as well as be an important representation of artists who broke away from abstract expressionism. After lunch, his wife showed up. "Oh, what's she doing here?" he complained to his boyfriend and partner, Nicola, as he became noticeably less animated. Since the conversation was in Italian, we weren't privy to what was being said. Soon after that Cy left, and we went for a walk in the walnut orchard.

We had some very itchy woolen bathing costumes from a circa 1900 pattern and badly fitted linen suits that a friend of ours had made for our trip. All the detail was perfect, except that they always looked wrinkled because our friend really had not mastered the art of tailoring. David's suit was a handkerchief linen—far too fine for a suit. It looked frumpy, and his undergarments (vintage one-piece) showed through. After dinner one evening David sat on a half-moon sofa with a fifties slipcover on it. When he discovered he had sat on a pen that broke on his suit and the sofa, Paola immediately asked for his pants and soaked them in milk, saying it would get the ink out of the fabric. McD tore off the slipcover to find an intact white-silk buttoned sofa from the thirties, the kind one would see in a Jean Harlow photograph. I looked up on the wall and saw a portrait of Paola's grandmother in a circular gold frame. She had marcelled platinum-blond hair with diamonds and pearls adorning her neck, hands, and head. We looked around at all the modernist paintings and figured out how the palazzo was originally decorated. The master portraitist Giovanni Boldini, John Singer Sargent's rival, had also painted her grandmother, though that portrait had been sold long ago. But Paola still had her grandmother's Dior New Look fashions from the late 1940s, which she wore with David's encouragement. She would walk us through the gates into town and show us the seventeenth-century buildings with endless rooms full of frescoes her family had given to the state.

We had gone to Naples for the first time the year before, in 1986, for our show with Lucio—*Fine Art Pictorial Guide of the Hudson River Valley*— which had sold out. They had warned us in Rome to be careful in Naples because of the crime there, but I never was bothered. I'd walk around at night and see someone breaking into a car. He'd nod at me and I would keep going. I loved visiting Naples, and where else could I have gotten a tiny bouquet wrapped in paper lace for a dollar to carry around all day. McD had high button shoes made but never picked them up. There was a square in the city center where the Catholic Church had knocked all the penises off the male statues and put fig leaves in their places, but the leaves had later been knocked off and the crotches painted blood red. The city had such a romantic and historic feel to it with all the crumbling buildings in ancient, narrow alleyways and tiny, modest cafés lit by fluorescent light serving delicious food.

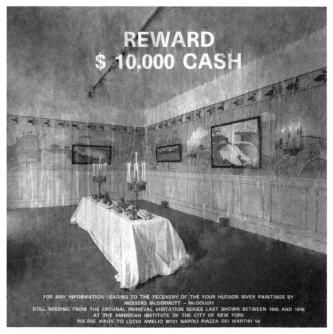

McD's playful ad for our show in Naples with Lucio Amelio

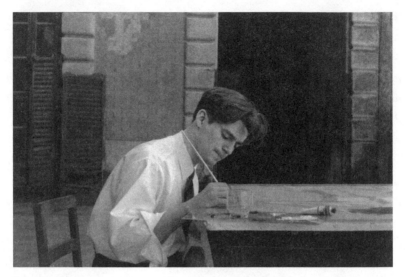

I am painting a Pompeiian-style portrait of Flavio di Bernardo on the terrace of his father's house, Villa Volpicelli.

I was in love with this city where we were supposed to go for two weeks but stayed five months. I gained forty pounds, so that on our return to New York, Jacqueline said it looked like I was melting.

On that first trip, one evening, walking back from our favorite restaurant, we came upon a group of *ragazzi* sitting on the hood of a car. They stopped us to speak in their broken English asking us about our clothes. One sexy type asked, "Do you like head?" Before I could say anything David broke in: "Hats! Well, yes—I love hats!" They all began to laugh, and we walked away. "You idiot," I whispered. "They said 'head,' not 'hats'! They wanted us." But Lucio had told us of the dangers of the Neapolitan streets, noting that there were many thieves preying on foreigners like us.

We stayed with Lucio in Villa Volpicelli, a private sixteenth-century villa built on ancient Roman ruins, with an Aragonese watchtower. The di Bernardo family's portraits by Warhol hung all over the house. Lucio told us that Andy had traded them for a suite of Bugatti furniture.

We painted on a huge terrace that had a jetty where all the boys in Speedos would lie sunning themselves. It was the summer of girls dressed like Madonna, with a big bow in the hair and a lot of bangle bracelets, and the boys with clean-cut barbershop looks riding Vespas. Lucio saw me looking them over and handed me binoculars. One day, outside Villa Volpicelli in Posillipo, near where Oscar Wilde stayed almost a century before, I saw a beautiful youth washing his hands in a work site above as he looked down on the street at me. I greeted him in my bad Italian. We had studied Italian with a former Fellini actor, Massimino Semprebene, who taught us formal Italian, but here they spoke a Neapolitan dialect. So our formal Italian was lost on the locals, who wanted to practice English conversation with us. I asked if he would pose for a painting. "How?" he asked. "*Nudo,*" I said. He agreed, and told me he would come by after work. We set a time and I went to tell McD, who was speaking with Chipa, the daughter of the family who owned the villa. She immediately stood up and screamed, "*No visitatori!* No visitors!" That evening she and her gorgeous brother, Flavio, came and waited with us at the gate. Soon a car full of *ragazzi* pulled up, including the beautiful youth. In Neapolitan dialect, a fight broke out between the family and the boys. A lot of hand waving and arguing ensued. I looked at the Caravaggio beauty and apologized with a frown. The five boys piled back into the small car and left. All I could think was that that would have been a very beautiful painting.

Another afternoon, outside the art shop, a charming, English-speaking male beauty stopped us on the street and asked if we were the artists with a show on. We said yes and took him to lunch. He came to our studio and flirted with us, but as I came closer to him, he drew back. When we returned the next year, with Bastian, I guess he was desperate about his life, and he aggressively went after me. Now it was my turn to draw back.

Lucio was nicknamed "the Queen of Naples," and rightfully so. He had established his gallery there in 1969 and showed such artists as Haring, Warhol, Twombly, Joseph Beuys, Gerhard Richter, Anselm Kiefer, and Robert Mapplethorpe. He was so well known in the town that no one harassed us, and perhaps it was also our wardrobe of old clothes. Everyone was friendly. Schoolchildren in old-fashioned pale-blue pin-

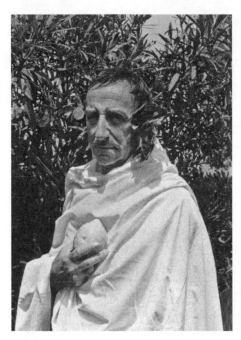

I took this picture of
Lucio Amelio in a bedsheet
and added a lemon and
laurel leaves from the garden in
Capri, posing him as a Roman
emperor. He was our dealer
for our only show in Naples.

afores and large red cravats would encircle us, loudly inquiring about
our look. People would call to us from windows and balconies while
hanging the wash. Lucio told us what restaurants to go to. At night he
would play the guitar and sing for us. He had made a record once and
had acted in four of Lina Wertmüller's films. He was a sort of local hero,
and people from restaurateurs to antique dealers called out to him from
their shops as he walked by. He had bought the German photographer
Baron Wilhelm von Gloeden's large nineteenth-century cameras, his
photographs of undraped youths, the glass negatives, postcards, and a
guest book with Oscar Wilde's signature in it. He had Joseph Beuys
draw on the postcards. I traded a painting for twelve of the photographs
and wished I had gotten some Beuys postcards. Mussolini's Fascist
police destroyed over two thousand of the baron's glass negatives.

After three days, we made our way to Capri and opened up the
apartment that we were renting from Paola. It had once belonged to
the nineteenth-century American symbolist artist Elihu Vedder, whose

paintings we admired. He designed the house and the furniture. When Paola's father died, the children took the house and made it into apartments. They tore out the grand staircase, and the furniture was stolen during the renovation, but it was a charming place and we were thrilled to be there. We slept in the front bedroom and Bastian was on a daybed in the living room. Our days were spent at the beach and in restaurants. We'd walk in our one-piece woolen bathing suits down the cliff to the rocky beach, having ascertained which had the least garbage floating in the water. Most days we'd meet Pat Hearn and Diego at the beach for lunch and a swim. We gossiped about George Condo, whom Pat had shown and lost to the Barbara Gladstone Gallery, which in turn lost him to Pace Gallery, where Julian showed, or about other art-world matters, such as who was sleeping with whom or the favorite show of the season. Kenny Scharf showed up, and we all went swimming in the Blue Grotto but left after plastic bags started to float in.

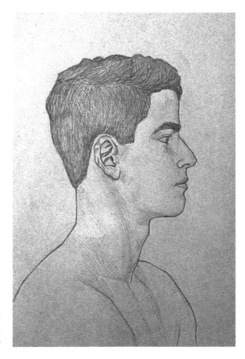

The drawing of Bastian
that I made in Capri,
summer 1987

One day Julian showed up in our Capri apartment. He had put on a lot of weight. "What are you doing here?" we asked. "Where's Jacqueline?"

"We're taking a break from each other. I'll see you later."

After he looked over our new paintings, I immediately went to the phone to call Jacqueline to find out what was happening. "We're just taking some time to ourselves," was all she said. I felt terrible for them. "How's Julian?" she asked.

"He seems sad and he's put on so much weight." "He's huge!" McD said, grabbing the receiver.

We saw Julian the next day at a restaurant and he said, "So you think I'm fat, huh?"

From Capri we would go back and forth on the ferry to Naples to buy art supplies and I started blocking out a few paintings, even though we were only there for a month. Bastian brought a modern camera that I used to take pictures of him. I also started a small canvas of him as a young Italian with laurel leaves on his head and a cloth draped to look like a toga. McD painted a Pompeiian border decoration around the sides.

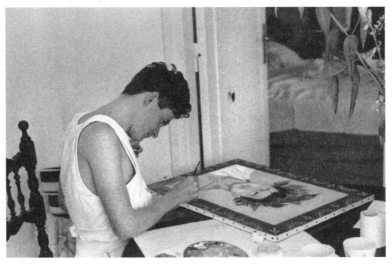

David painting the trim on Bastian's portrait which I had just painted

In a nod to the Italian futurist movement, we made a painting that read "Dandyismo" with Robert Delaunay sort-of-abstract shapes and letters floating around it, like our earlier painting *A Friend of Dorothy*. Paola came to visit and collect the rent. We'd never even asked what the rent was. It was four thousand for the month, which we didn't have. Luckily, on a shelf she saw two little paintings I had just made: one of Vesuvius, with a question mark of smoke rising out of it, and another of a modernist wheel. Lucio was always good for financial advances. Like the other dealers we had, he liked the idea of a group deal, buying all we made. Since the days were very relaxing and Bastian did nothing but read, I'd get him to pose for paintings and marveled at his youth and beauty. One evening we went with Diego and Pat to a party given by the Hamburg art dealer Ascan Crone. His guest was the writer Gary Indiana, who at the time wrote an art column for *The Village Voice*, in which he called us the "Tupperware Gilbert and George," after the English art duo. I didn't know who they were when I started working with David; but one day early on, when we were walking around the East Village in our summer whites, a man came up to us and asked, "Are you Gilbert and George?" I replied, "No. My name's Peter." Gary also wrote that *A Friend of Dorothy* should have been the cover of the 1987 Biennial catalog.

After dinner Diego, Pat, and the three of us left the party. We walked home talking animatedly with a silent, rigid Bastian. Once we were back home, he let out his disgust for the conversation and the guests, "You're all nothing but a bunch of gossips living in an art bubble." Bastian hated all our friends and loathed the art world. His snobbery became vindictive. "They're idiots," he'd say. "And those dealers take a 50 percent commission and treat you with no respect unless you make them money!"

Unfortunately, soon enough Bastian had David's ear on most matters. They fit together like peas in a pod, intellectually. They didn't need anyone else. At first it didn't bother me, because Bastian was more talkative than I was and I lived mostly in my head. McD was in awe of Bastian's brains and beauty. David didn't like men his own age: "They have too many problems and are set in their ways. I like to influence whom I'm interested in romantically." They were happy in their discussion of books, David's theories, and many historical topics. Bastian sat at McD's feet to learn about detachable collars, decorating, and his views of the world. Whenever their antics—and there were many—got them in trouble, I'd boil into a rage. They'd look at me in shock and tell me that I needed to calm down. "We're Aquarians, Peter," McD would spout, "and you're a Cancer. We're intellectual—you are emotional." That made me even more livid.

Over the years McD would win most of our fights because he threatened me with a burning-red face with veins popping. "I know how to fight!" he'd warn me. "I'll tear the whole house down! So, if you want to start something, I'll finish it!" And I knew he would. In the past, he

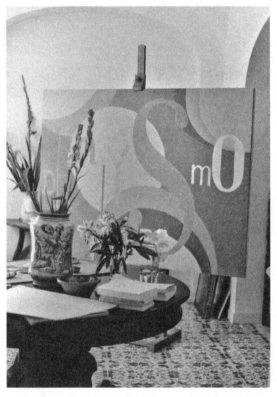

The sitting room in Paola's house in Capri with our *Dandyismo* on the easel

had slashed and kicked in paintings, thrown chairs into mirrors, and overturned fully set tables. Or vases would fly across the room. His rants and rages were embedded in my memory. I knew what could happen, so I'd back off, as there was no winning an argument. I knew he had no boundaries when he threatened me. I'd seen him at his worst before, and I'd go silent.

Near the end of our stay Lucio came by to look at the paintings. He asked Diego if he should buy them and Diego gave his approval. So Lucio bought everything except Bastian's portrait, which we kept. We closed up the house, making our way to the ferry to Naples with a wad of cash.

In Rome we stayed at the Grand Hotel Plaza, which had a large marble lion at the end of the main interior staircase. Our rooms hadn't been changed since the turn of the century. Everything was intact, especially the bath. It was exactly what we had hoped for. We had breakfast in the vast restaurant in the hotel, with its red flocked walls and plush velvet drapery. Our continental breakfast came with a cup of coffee and a muffin—most unfortunately, in plastic wrapping.

When we returned to Manhattan, McD suggested we go to Hudson to stay with his mentor, and Bastian could stop off and then continue farther upstate, where he was from. After Capri, Bastian's mood seemed to change, and he became distant. We thought the party had ended and we'd never meet again. We went back to our place on Avenue C, where McD had had the metal doors torn out, and was having them replaced with handmade mahogany doors and reproduction box locks with brass keys. Then we went to see Massimo.

14

t's all bubbles and stripes now!" Massimo cried. "You should have stayed in Italy!" Meaning the mood had changed and the collectors were looking for less figurative and more minimalist and modern-looking artwork. It was nicknamed "neo-geo"—new geometric.

McD and Massimo argued a lot. It was always about David's need for more money. After our first show he went to Massimo to ask for money again. Massimo went into a rage, insulting him. There was a painting of ours in the gallery and Massimo screamed, "Look at your painting—it looks like shit!" I saw McD's face twitch and grow red. He went over to the painting and kicked a hole in it and screamed, "*Now* it looks like shit!" I gasped as Massimo slumped onto his desk with a thunderous cry and McD stormed out of the gallery.

A letter came in the mail from Bastian. We were surprised that he wrote us. He had left in such a state that we didn't expect ever to see or hear from him again—and besides, he was finishing off his last year at prep school. But this letter was apologetic and grateful for the trip to Italy. Years later he found and destroyed all his letters to us.

David went to the desk and wrote one of his beautiful letters with a nib pen and inkwell, sealing it with wax and a pressed stamp. McD's letters were as beautiful as a painting, well written and dated in the past with an old stamp. In a week Bastian's second letter came, followed by a phone call. I had convinced McD we needed a phone. We bought a bell box and a candlestick telephone from the twenties that we kept on a table in the hallway. Bastian was calling to say he was quitting school in his senior year. David was adamant that he stay and finish his last year of the scholarship. But Bastian was determined to leave. After a bit of back-and-forth he asked if he could come and stay with us.

I still think of that moment when he came up to me at the reception after our show in New England and spoke to me. What a fool I was to fall for his youth and beauty and his green eyes! I was smitten at first, as he was attractive, intelligent, and well-read, spoke a few languages, and seemed truly interested in us. But later something seemed sour in the soup.

I do not recommend a ménage à trois. One person is always left out, and that one was me. Bastian's strengths played to my insecurities. I had always thought of myself as an idiot. I had barely graduated from high school, but in our early days in Hudson, David built up my self-confidence. Now, with Bastian at his side, my longtime partner seemed less interested in me, and Bastian became McD's acolyte. McD wanted twelve boyfriends, "just like Jesus," he'd say. One would be for writing projects (Bastian), one for painting (me?), one for filmmaking, and so on. McD would always try to add another name to the Messrs. McDermott & McGough, "just like a law firm." But I wasn't having it. I worked too hard, and I wasn't going to add on the name of his latest crush.

Once Bastian was living with us, if David went after a new "apostle" Bastian punished him by ignoring him or leaving for hours. One day after a fight Bastian left the house. His suitcase was gone, and he wasn't around. David thought he'd gone to his mother's, so we called her. Bastian's mother was the ultimate WASP, a member of the Daughters of the American Revolution in L.L.Bean and madras skirts and headbands. I was a bit embarrassed that I called because she hadn't heard from him and now was worried. I decided to go to Grand Central to look for him, thinking he might try to catch the train for upstate. I waited, but he didn't appear. I just thought maybe I should call the house in case he was there and sure enough, he was. He had hidden his suitcase under the bed skirt and gone for a walk. When I returned to Avenue C, Bastian was furious at me for calling his mother, but I reprimanded him for pulling such a prank.

Bastian fit perfectly into vintage clothing, since he was short. "People in the past were much smaller," McD would say. David liked to dress him up like a doll, buying him any clothes he wanted, from a gray linen 1920s suit to a French military uniform from the 1840s—and it didn't stop there. Somehow the scenario felt deeply familiar: when I moved in with David, I had been his doll, too.

Our strategy of positivity from *The Game of Life* slowly descended the staircase and went out the front door. In its place was Bastian's bitter elitist attitude. With his loathing of the art-world gatherings and the gay life we led, he pushed many of our friends away. Slowly I realized that our young enchanter's divide-and-conquer scheme had begun to destroy my life with McD. Bastian's grip on McD was extremely strong, as he held him with scattered sexual favors. And soon Bastian's appetite for acquisition matched David's own.

As a country place, we had rented a large eighteenth-century house outside of Rhinebeck, New York, with the original carved fireplaces and painted floors. Then one weekend in Manhattan, McD and Bastian with some visiting friends from Vienna took a bus to Atlantic City to see a car show. They came back with a 1913 Model T Ford convertible with wooden wheels. Since both McD and I were uninterested in driving, Bastian was a perfect housemate to take over cars and, later, the horses.

Black Monday, October 19, 1987, was the day the stock market crashed. We didn't have a television or radio and we hardly ever looked at newspapers, since McD liked to get his news from hearsay and gossip. I knew

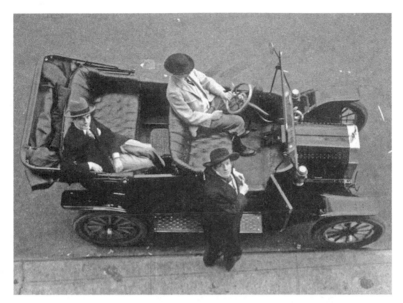

The 1913 Model T with Bastian at the wheel, David in a Hasidic hat, and me in the backseat

of the crash, but I didn't think it would affect the art world or us. Our work was still selling well, and we had future exhibitions lined up. We had never saved a penny, however. In addition to the Model T we had bought a 1925 Model A truck that didn't work and a pile of antiques. We had a big staff—as many as fourteen people which included a chef preparing lunches at one point. There were also three horses, handmade saddles, boots, wagons, three properties, three automobiles, fancy restaurants like the Odeon, Bar Pitti, and Il Cantinori, and parties and many bills that we didn't pay.

Massimo had been very successful, and in 1988 he had taken a large space in SoHo and asked us to do a show. We usually ate in a restaurant on Avenue A that had paper tablecloths and crayons, so we decided to do a drawing show of our lives in crayon and make a large painting, *Trying to Get There,* ten feet long, of the climb to fame, after an image from the twenties we found in Kenneth Anger's *Hollywood Babylon.* With the show up, David wanted Massimo to raise the price of the large painting by five thousand dollars, but Massimo felt that would be too much to ask at the time. He had rented the Mr Chow restaurant on Fifty-Seventh Street for the dinner after the opening, and when they asked David to sing, as he usually did, he declined. The disagreement over the price led to another big fight between them, and we parted ways. Lucio dropped us soon after. Julian ran into Lucio and asked why he didn't pay us the money he owed us. That ended up with Lucio screaming at me in front of an art-fair crowd of gossipmongers and onlookers. Then his secretary sent us the remaining money he owed. So now we had no dealer. I took to my bed for a month. We were offered representation with a good dealer in SoHo, but I turned them down since I felt McD would clash with them, too. I loved Massimo. He was so good to us, such a sweet and crazy person. He had a very funny way of speaking. In his broken English he'd utter sentences like "Don't raise my voice to me!" and "How dare you are!" or, if he was attracted to someone, he "had a hard one on!" He would do hysterical impersonations of art-world types that kept us in stitches. But the now defunct *Arts Magazine* gave us a scathing full-page review of the crayon drawings, calling us in the first paragraph "adolescent narcissists," and in the last noting our "self-promotional inconsequential narcissism." In a future review of our photography they called us fetishists. At the time I was crushed.

Through Diego we had met the art dealer Howard Read, a kinetic man with a Roman-coin profile who knew everything about photography, from Daguerre to Mapplethorpe. They both suggested we take up photography, saying it would go well with our work. Neither David nor I had studied cameras or how they worked. One Sunday, on one of our ritualistic visits to the flea market, we bought a wooden camera from 1910. It had its original brass lens and wooden film holders for an eight-by-ten-inch image. Later we found a larger eleven-by-fourteen-inch camera with its wooden tripod.

McD's intensity meant everything had to be perfect, down to the block of ice in the wooden icebox, which he would pick up with large cast-iron tongs and put in his bicycle basket to bring home as it dripped onto his pant leg. There was an enamel drip pan below the icebox that caught the melting water and had to be emptied periodically. David liked to show it off to guests as if it were the latest invention.

I started taking pictures of Bastian, David, and Jacqueline and her children Lola and Stella, as well as still lives. We brought the black-and-white contact sheets (each image was eight by ten) to Howard's gallery. Howard said they were nice but wanted to see them printed. Through James Wheeler, the photography assistant we all had a crush on, we started with a cyanotype process from the nineteenth century, which gives a bluish hue to the photograph, and the only materials needed are ammonia, water, and cyan. After a few tries we finally had the cyan images that we wanted. We brought the blue pictures to Howard who loved them and asked if he could hold on to them for

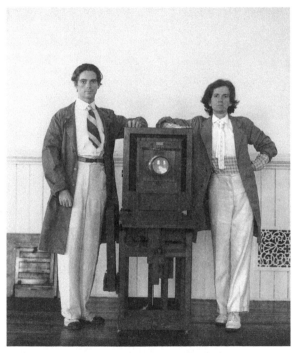

Posing in our studio at the Kings County Savings Bank in Williamsburg with the camera we used for our first show at the Robert Miller Gallery

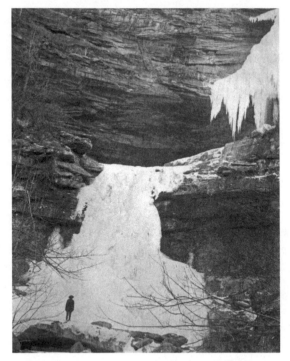

Travel to the Bottom of the Earth, 1907/1988:
Our 8 x 10 cyanotype photograph of the frozen
Kaaterskill Falls, with David at the bottom

the weekend. The following Tuesday he called and offered us a show uptown on Fifty-Seventh Street in the smaller room of the Robert Miller Gallery.

We went on taking pictures. We climbed down an icy path to photograph the frozen Kaaterskill Falls with McD at the bottom in a large-brimmed beaver hat we bought from a Hasidic shop in Williamsburg. We made still lives in Rhinebeck, and I asked Bastian to pose naked after an Ingres painting, and also used other Ingres paintings as inspiration for posing the studio assistants. Making a photographic image seemed so much easier than painting: the image was almost immediate.

After Julian left his studio on Twentieth Street, we asked Jacqueline if we could use it since Ross Bleckner wanted his White Street studio. We moved in all of our paint, canvases, and cameras.

In a discussion with Howard, he happened to mention he had sold a Mapplethorpe to a collector who took the image out of the artist's frame and discarded the frame. We took this as a warning, and we designed our frames to have wavy reproduction glass with tiny flaws and bubbles to give them an original look. McD came up with the idea of having a label printed that read, "The Temple of Photographic Art, 18__," which would be glued on the back so no one could throw out the frame, as it was part of the artwork. In his flowery hand McD would sign our names, the name of the photograph, and the date 1907, since we felt the photographs looked like they came from that period.

We planned an evening at the Twentieth Street studio and asked Fred Hughes, who arrived with the lawyer Ed Hayes and Julian. We had become very friendly with the impeccably dressed Fred after Andy died. Fred was suffering from MS and getting weaker by the month, but later, he generously gave Bastian his twenty-first-birthday party at his amazing townhouse up on Lexington Avenue for just the four of us—the invitation demanded full dress tails. In Julian's old studio we had pinned the blue images to the wall and went through them with Julian, removing what we thought wouldn't work. Ed Hayes stood by the window, looking at a fortune-teller's neon sign, and mumbled something about Gypsies.

The attention we received for the show, which John Cheim curated in 1989, was colossal. It was also the 150th anniversary of the invention of the photograph, so we were included in many shows because of that. Harry Lunn, the art dealer who championed such photographers as Walker Evans, Diane Arbus, Robert Frank, and Robert Mapplethorpe and was called "the Godfather of Photography," bought half of our show.

We felt that our paintings expressed our theories on time, homo-eroticism, and history while the new photographs were a record of our lives. We also wanted the photographs to look, to the untrained eye, like period images. With McD's intense obsession with making sure he lived in his time machine, I could turn the camera anywhere on our private lives and get an interesting image. And that's how we made our first show. It sold out three times over with our edition of only three images each. Bastian, with his affection for language, wrote the titles for the images such as *The Achievement of Sublimity Through the Renunciation of Temporality* and *Congregation of Illumination* and *Tory Fecundity*.

Since the photographs were selling, Howard asked for new and larger images. So we looked for a mammoth plate camera. We traded a painting for a large old camera from photographer Timothy Greenfield-Sanders who took photographs of downtown artists and other well-known figures. We had the old lens, but we had to make a new front and film holders, and it was quite difficult to maneuver the large holders. The film they held was twenty-four by twenty inches. Since the lens didn't have a cap, I used an old battered bowler hat and would count "One . . . two . . . three" as the sitter held still. "Don't blink!" I'd call out.

Even with the vast number of photographs Howard sold each year we always seemed to be broke. One day we sold a hundred grand's worth of paintings—the equivalent of $214,000 now. That was mostly gone in three days. Adding to his many possessions, McD had bought a large navy 1930 Graham-Paige automobile. It had a moss-colored mohair interior with a green silk shade in the rear window complete with a tassel. A cut-glass bud vase was screwed into the side of the door on the right. Since it was not heated, it had a blanket bar on which we kept a heavy throw, like what we used in the Model T. It was very otherworldly sitting in the back as David and Bastian sat in the front: I could stare out the window and dream.

One morning in Rhinebeck I was picking the orange lilies that covered the front lawn when Bastian and David ran out and jumped into the Model T with two hunting dogs and a wagon wheel. They yelled they'd be going for a ride and taking the wagon wheel to the Amish, who'd repair it. I didn't pay much attention because they were always up to something. McD was a truly adventurous person. I went about my day and waited for them to return for lunch. Then I waited for dinner. Still no show. I went to bed unable to call them and with no call from them. The next day was nearing dusk when they finally showed up in the drive.

"Where the hell have you been?" I shouted.

"We went to Canada!"

They would often drive the Model T to and from the city using the back roads since the car went too slowly for the highway; the trip took six hours instead of two. I would usually take the train and meet them, but once I rode with them from the city to Rhinebeck. By this time, the convertible top wouldn't go up, and since it was raining part of the way, I opened an umbrella. Then the sun came out and we were almost home. Just as we were flying along, Bastian made a sharp turn onto the road where the house was. One of the wooden wheels that held the white tires cracked and fell off and the car lurched forward. I was seated in the back, and suddenly I was flying over Bastian and David toward the road. I had heard how in accidents people report that time moves at a different pace. Now I could confirm that: everything felt like it was in slow motion as I looked down on Bastian and McD seated below me. In an instant I fell facedown onto the macadam road just off a two-lane highway only yards away from the accident. Sprawled on my chest, I was stunned but not knocked out. My first thought on seeing my recently purchased nineteenth-century silver pocket watch, facedown too, with its key attached to its chain was that it would be totally ruined. I reached out and turned it over to find it in pristine condition. I pulled myself up to see a shocked McD. A station wagon stopped and a man and woman jumped out and hurried over to me: "We have to get you to a hospital!"

I screamed, "Leave me alone—I'm a Christian Scientist! Go away!"

"I was just trying to help!" the man barked, as he and his wife went back to their car. I turned and saw our car behind him in a ditch, with the front smashed and the broken wooden wheel that flew off a few feet away. At first I burst into tears, then rage pushed aside the tears and I became furious. "I could have been killed! What the fuck is wrong with you two!" The years of swallowing my fury about them was coming to a head. McD came up to me and said, "You seem all right. Why don't you walk up the street and take a bath, that will calm you down."

"*Calm down?!*" I screamed. "I'm not interested in fucking calming down! I am so sick of the two of you and your fucking hijinks! I could have been killed!" Bastian was standing across the street in silence. I pushed by and walked up the road till I reached the house, lamenting my mad relationships. An hour later they returned and David came into my room to check on me. I was still shaken but had calmed myself.

"We had to wait for a truck to take the car to a repair shop."

I didn't answer. I just looked at him.

"Too bad we didn't have our camera here. It would have made a great photo."

I didn't reply as I turned to face the other way.

Over the next day I kept silent and mostly continued reading in my room. Bastian milled about the house avoiding me and never came over to discuss what had happened.

Julian was looking for a studio, and one day when McD was going over the Williamsburg Bridge, he saw a rental sign on an old bank built in the 1860s French Second Empire style. We went to look at it with Julian, but he didn't want to be so far from Manhattan, and Williamsburg seemed very far away at that time. Then McD said we should take it as our studio. I objected to yet another expense but McD was determined. The top two floors were available (a new bank had moved into the ground-floor space, which still had its original bank booths), twenty-five hundred square feet each. The toilets hadn't been changed since 1900, and in the very top of the building was an old room with faded original wallpaper where we could see the outlines of framed images taken down long ago. We rented the two floors, used the lower one as our studio, and painted the walls light blue; the top floor, with twenty-three-foot ceilings, was our photography studio, which we painted a dark orange.

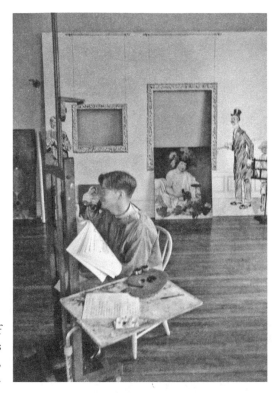

I'm painting in one of our studios in the Kings County Savings Bank, Williamsburg, Brooklyn.

Later the bank went under and we took the street floor, too. We rented all three floors for eight thousand a month. In addition, we had the rent on our apartment on Avenue C and the house upstate. Next, McD went on a spending spree to decorate the three floors of the bank building. He bought a huge conference table and chairs for the ground floor, but we already had quite a lot of furniture from various storage spaces. All our costumes and period clothes went up to the photo studio, where we made a painted backdrop for doing portraits. We had met Bernard-Ruiz Picasso, the artist's grandson, a handsome Spaniard, who asked us to take a photograph of him for his grandmother. We set about dressing him in a high starched collar and a red striped shirt with a white bow tie. He had the most amazing profile. I used the mammoth plate camera as well as the eleven-by-fourteen one to do the portraits. A young southerner, David Lee Jones, was our assistant then. He helped with the settings on the camera and set up our dark room with a massive wooden sink to print the large negatives and a drying rack. We had to special-order the film from Kodak for the mammoth plate camera. They would make it if we ordered it in bulk. It was so expensive we split the cost with photographer Adam Fuss, who showed us how to work our large-negative wooden camera.

The Flemings, John Patrick and Walter, had a house up in the Catskills. They told us about a property we had to buy in Oak Hill, the next town over. We went to look at it with them, peeked into the eighteenth-century windows, and fell in love with the place.

It was a brick house from 1790 that had a working hand pump by the side of the kitchen as its only source of water, a large 1880s general store next to it, and an apartment with original wallpaper. The store that stood there was tacked onto the back with large barns behind it and a two-seater outhouse that had a wallpapered interior and a drawer that, when full, you could pull out and empty. Neither building had

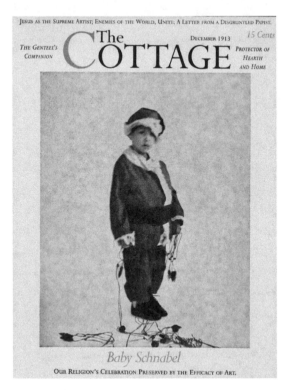

We remade McD's pamphlet *The Cottage* into an actual typeset magazine to keep Bastian occupied. We made Vito Schnabel Baby Santa.

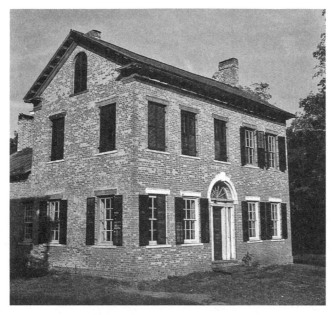

The outside of our Oak Hill house

been modernized. Behind was a running creek. We saw all this after we made an appointment with the elderly real-estate woman. She told us she used to own it and that it had been empty for decades. We had to restrain ourselves when she told us the store was intact when she bought it a decade before, with all its original merchandise, down to the wooden barrels that were packed with excelsior to keep the early kerosene lamps from breaking. But she had turned it into an antiques store and sold everything piecemeal. Afterwards, McD said it took great control for him not to start screaming at her for wrecking the store's original condition.

We didn't act fast enough and the house was sold. A few years later, however, it came on the market again, and since we had just sold a group of paintings we bought the property. We set up a balloon payment so we didn't have to put down as much money and the former owner held the mortgage. After moving in, we began a deeper headway into the past through Bastian's passion for horses.

Quite a lot of money was coming in with sales of our photographs and paintings. We had never experienced anything like it. We bought Bastian two Morgan horses that he kept behind the house after building a fenced-in area for them. Then there was all the custom tack that was needed along with the hay, the grains, the blacksmith, and the vets. I used an old shed in back as a painting studio. I couldn't use the barns because we had just bought a two-seated carriage, a surrey, and a wooden omnibus with a painted side that sat eighteen.

We made another trip to Williamsburg, Virginia, and bought a pile of copper pots, wooden buckets with rope handles, kitchen ladles, and other spoons. We also brought locks of our long hair to have eighteenth-century wigs made. We returned to the Catskills with everything we had gotten. McD had bought two tin washtubs connected by a wooden table for one of his favorite pastimes: laundry. He'd wash, then rinse, our clothes and put them through a wringer and dry them on a line.

McD would always say, "I know how to spend money." He had great taste in objects and furniture and could spot them with ease, but he never learned the art of saving. He bragged that he never wasted money on alcohol and drugs, "so I don't feel guilty spending it on antiques." He still shaves with a straight-edge razor. He had so many interests in each century and their decades that he started to shop even more. For the apartment on Avenue C, the furniture was from 1835 to 1865; the eighteenth-century house in Oak Hill was early American, 1750–1820; and the studio in Williamsburg was late nineteenth century to 1930. He was always buying or picking up broken antiques in the street and having them repaired. He found a wicker-furniture repairman upstate and brought all the worn-out chairs and little tables to him. He was creating his fantasy, stating, "This is my real art." He was a natural installation artist.

Bastian bought a child's old wooden wagon. He had harnesses made for the two hunting dogs we had bought him—a Springer and a Brittany spaniel. He hooked them up to the wagon, and we then put our two miniature dachshunds in the back. When we arrived at the Williamsburg Bridge, the dogs became excited as David, Bastian, and I ran alongside. Sometimes Bastian would jump in for a ride.

In the late 1980s, *House & Garden* contacted us to come by and meet the then editor-in-chief, Anna Wintour. She wanted to do a story on Avenue C, but we had to decline because *Vanity Fair* had already asked to do a story on Avenue C and the way we dressed. The apartment was not papered, so we went to Albany and bought up the last remaining rolls of the 1930s Victorian revival wallpapers we were interested in. We stopped in at Louis Bowen, which made paper, and asked for the paper ceiling borders for the rooms. Weeks went into hiring a paper hanger and then our making the endless final touches on the house. When we had finished, we asked Justin Hoag to come over and decorate the tables with our etched compote glassware and other Victorian dishes for the article. He went about building beautiful pyramids of fruit, garlanded the house with fir-tree branches, and put up a Christmas tree and decorated it with our extensive collection of nineteenth-century ornaments and candle holders. We asked Julian's former girlfriend Jean Kalina to come over to take the pictures for the magazine. David, Bastian, Justin, and I dressed up in black top hats, and we were joined by our friend Simon Bowden, who was visiting from London, as Jean photographed us holding hands and dancing around the Christmas tree. She took many beautiful pictures, but soon *Vanity Fair* called and said they were canceling the shoot because they wanted to do a bigger story on Nancy and Ronald Reagan, who were on the cover. We were not pleased but consoled ourselves by realizing the walls were papered and our home was finished. Lucio came in from Naples and we invited him for tea. When he arrived, he couldn't get over the splendor of it all.

The way we dressed and lived was an editorial dream for interior magazines. The art magazines could be critical. They'd start a review of a show of ours by calling us dandies. By the end of the review some would go in for the kill: we were creating "a sort of precocious dandyism that is all the more impressive for its determination not to be taken too seriously. By wanting to be seen only as sexy eccentrics with perfect party manners, they make smart bids for superstardom by convincingly playing their parts." David is an eccentric, but neither of us ever thought of ourselves as sexy, and we surely didn't have perfect party manners. One reviewer even criticized us for eating in restaurants. Or another said that, "they even wear painters' smocks and use easels and palettes, like artists in an opera." I thought that was very funny. We considered ourselves not dandies but modern artists making a living performance about time.

15

David's high-school friend from New Jersey, Roseanne, married Michael Burlingham, who was part of the Tiffany family. Michael didn't inherit money, only a trunk with letters from important people of the last century, like Teddy Roosevelt. There was also a scrapbook that included press clippings on Louis Comfort Tiffany's 1913 Egyptian Fête which was held in the enormous fourth-floor studio at Tiffany's when it was on Madison and Forty-Fifth Street. The French sculptor Francis Tonetti created a scene of a terrace in the city of Alexandria overlooking the Mediterranean, with the German actress Hedwiga Reicher playing Cleopatra and Ruth St. Denis dancing. There was a craze then called Egyptomania, dating back to the 1869 opening of the Suez Canal.

McD became inspired to have a fête of our own. His first step was to have the invitation copied from Tiffany's original. It was on parchment paper, rolled and tied in a string, sealed with wax, and hand-delivered around town. The invitation stated: "Dress in the time of Cleopatra."

We hired a friend who was a seven-foot-tall black man to be the guard at the door of our studio in the bank in Williamsburg and stand between two urns with fire flaming out of them. They were actually

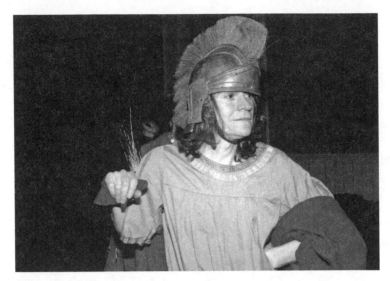

David in a helmet from James Nares's film *Rome '78* at the Egyptian
fête we gave at our studios in the Kings County Savings Bank

two city garbage cans with wood from the street that we doused with
lighter fluid. You could do anything in that neighborhood then, just
like in Alphabet City. We had a man in a white robe reading from the
Koran in the echoing hallway as the visitors arrived, but we soon had to
ask him to leave because he was groping the scantily clad female guests.
We copied eight outfits that Michael had from the original fête for our
guests who came without costume. On the second floor we had an Arab
band with a belly dancer as four peacocks walked freely between ropes
that made a fence around the columns.

Upstairs was an eighteen-piece orchestra that played popular dance
music from the 1910s. I was dressed as the Indian goddess Lakshmi, in
scraps of Indian fabrics, and McD wore a Roman helmet, shield, and
leg guards from his movie *Rome '78*; he kind of resembled the space-
man from Bugs Bunny cartoons. Jacqueline Schnabel came dressed
as Cleopatra, wearing a necklace and headdress and a flowing, silk
lime-green gown. We served Middle Eastern food to guests lounging on
blankets and pillows. Afterwards David and I climbed up the steps to
a stagelike wooden platform with an Egyptian backdrop of the Sphinx

and the Pyramids as Jacqueline was carried through the crowd on a wheelless rickshaw by two scantily dressed musclemen to join us on the stage. We then had the party revelers form a line, and bow as they were introduced to us. And of course there was no alcohol, to the chagrin of the guests. Some ran across the street to Peter Luger's restaurant in their costumes to load up on booze. We spent twenty thousand dollars on the evening. That night in our studio it was 1990, 1913, and 40 BC all at the same time. It was a joyful evening, in the midst of a crack epidemic and AIDS. The future seemed bleak, and the party was a celebration in spite of it all.

Many guests brought cameras but we had an assistant use an eight-by-ten vintage camera to make portraits of the guests. Bastian didn't show up in my images because he sat against the wall canoodling with a young lady friend. Afterwards, from the guests' modern flash-camera shots, the party looked like it was a high-school drama production. But under the candlelight it had a warm, cozy, romantic feel. McD still had his relationship with Bastian, and maybe I just didn't get along with this pale Narcissus because I found him unkind. McD, despite his nuttiness and temper tantrums, was still a kind person. He had a reputation for being unhinged, but would be unexpectedly kind to people he did not know and always generous with friends who needed help. Bastian I found pompous: he'd look in the mirror and say, "Don't you ever die!" and laugh. I also hated his right-wing politics and his selective homophobia.

McD and I really weren't drinkers unless it was expensive wine and someone else paid. But Bastian liked his spirits and would often come home tipsy. David had a way of folding socks that he saw in an old magazine. He would fold them into little flat cakes and line them up by color in a drawer. One evening on Avenue C, a boozed-up Bastian came stumbling into his room, opened the sock drawer, and threw up in it before passing out in bed. At the rental we had outside Rhinebeck from 1978 to 1980, the owner had an apartment in the basement. One day she came upstairs and accused us of drinking all her liquor. McD reprimanded her: we were temperate and he hated booze. I was in my

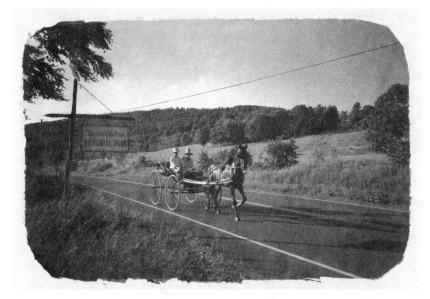

Bastian and David wearing straw top hats in our buggy with the famous wild stallion in Oak Hill

room and Bastian came in and lay down on the bed next to me. I could tell he was drunk and he smelled of it. Since we didn't keep liquor in the house, I guessed where he'd found it. He snuggled up against me and kissed me passionately. I pushed him away. I couldn't take this intruder in my house any longer. I wanted him out. But he and David were bound together. He'd sleep in David's bed, and in the morning I'd find them entwined and sound asleep. It seemed sad that most discussions of our life had to include this kid who so hated the world that supported us all.

Bastian preferred the country life, but I liked our artistic circle of friends in New York, so we kept his horse and carriage in Prospect Park. McD and he would hitch up the horse and drive around Brooklyn with kids running after them cheering. Bastian even rode a horse over the Williamsburg Bridge to an opening in Manhattan, dressed in his red hunt coat.

The horse was a beautiful stallion that we had bought upstate. One day I had been in bed reading, ensconced in the cloud of our feather mattress, and Bastian joined me to cuddle and seduce. Afterwards, in the sweetest voice, he asked if I would give him five thousand dollars to buy the stallion. We already had two Morgan horses, but being a chump, I wrote the check. That weekend we all went to the farm that was selling the stallion. It was a magnificent creature, black with a beautiful full mane and tail. An old man said that the horse was untrainable and a wild beast. But that didn't derail Bastian. He had the farmer tie the horse to a fence while he put his handmade saddle on the stallion and got on. As the horse took off with him on it, Bastian—who was pint-sized anyway—looked like a small child on the snorting and frantic steed. To my amazement, in less than an hour he had that horse riding backwards and sideways. It was interesting to watch him hold the attention of the group that now was his audience. The old men and the farmer could not believe this beast was tamed.

After buying Oak Hill, David rented a magnificent early-eighteenth-century stone house on a highway an hour away. It still had a shadow of

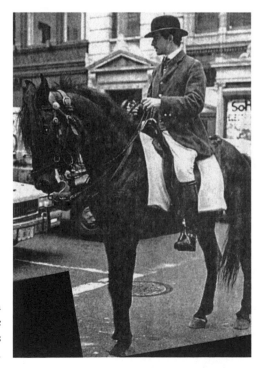

Bastian rode the stallion over the Williamsburg Bridge to Michael O'Donoghue's show at the Cable Building.

crossed swords over the mantel. The house was resplendently original, but now we had another rent and also a mortgage to pay. We had sent Bastian down south to Virginia to train with a horseman who drove carriages in a city park. Cowboy Bob (I'm changing the name to protect the guilty) knew a lot about horses and guns; he had about thirty weapons in his house. As McD confirmed for me later, following one visit, I could tell Cowboy Bob didn't care for me—and likewise. He was a braggard, pompous, and also a conspiracy theorist. He wasn't stupid, though—he was very intelligent. He always wore the same khaki army outfit with a cowboy hat, and had a stinky cigar tucked under his mustache. He thought I was a "big fag," as McD often repeated to me, but somehow he didn't feel the same way about Bastian and David. I didn't care, I considered myself a walking advertisement for an old-fashioned homosexual. With Bob one could hardly get a word in, he was such an overbearing presence. And now, with David, Bastian, and Bob all speaking over one another, there was no room for me.

In the spring of 1990 we were getting ready for a booth at Chicago's art fair with our new dealers, Sperone Westwater. Bruno Bischofberger had asked Gian Enzo Sperone, a handsome, immaculately dressed Italian who partnered with Angela Westwater, a thin wisp of a blonde who had been in the art world since the early seventies, to exhibit our paintings. For our booth, we went about making backdrops that were copies of the interior and exterior of the bank studio, then hung our paintings over the backdrops. We rented an antique table and chairs and a large Persian carpet to cover the industrial one. The booth was a sold-out success, and we received many compliments as being "best in show." In November we were to have our first show with Sperone Westwater in SoHo. McD had come up with the idea that each painting would be housed in a white military-styled tent with a twenty-five-cent charge to get inside—if you didn't have the invitation with free tickets. The card read, "Sperone Westwater—Purveyors of High Class Art. Want

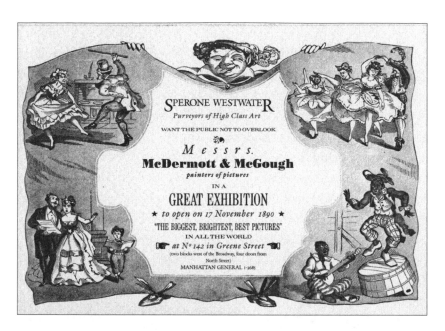

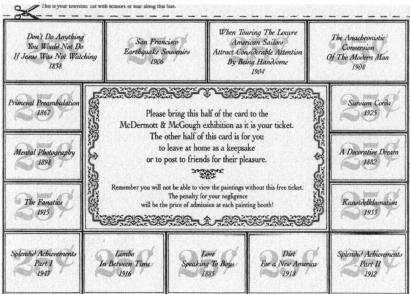

McDermott designed the invitation for our first show at Sperone Westwater.

the public not to overlook Messrs. McDermott & McGough painters of pictures in a GREAT EXHIBITION. The Biggest, Brightest, Best Pictures." I did find McD's humor very funny. Angela objected that the tents wouldn't be able to protect the paintings, which couldn't be seen by the person at the reception desk. But McD was adamant in his vision and angry at her refusal to cooperate. The evening of our opening he said he wasn't going to the show. His mentor was there from upstate. I begged him to get dressed and come with me. I did not want to get into a fight. My pleading was ignored. The mentor then took an old tome from the bookshelf and said, "Let's open the Bible to see what Jesus wants." At this point I was ready to do anything. I understood McD's anger that his vision had been thwarted, but this last-minute stubbornness was too much for me. Finally, McD listened to his mentor as he closed his eyes, put his finger on a page in the Bible, and announced that Jesus said McD should go to the opening. We arrived just as the opening was ending and Vivian was on her way out. The show sold well, but we received very mixed reviews. The *Times* gave it a decent-sized review with an image, but the last paragraph was a slap in the face. Some reviewers didn't know what to think of us. Over the years we were accused of: making up our names, being racist, sexist, anti-Semitic, Nazis, even homophobic (?)—and, of course, fakes and poseurs.

In 1991 our photography was included in another Whitney Biennial. The curator and publisher Raymond Foye, whom I knew through Allen Ginsberg and Diego, gave us a French book from the nineteenth century called *Les Récréations scientifiques,* full of images illustrating how objects in the home could have other uses. One example was to tie a string around the handle of a large serving spoon and hold the ends of the string in each ear and bang the spoon on a table top. The effect would sound like church bells. This was very useful for saving a boring dinner. We copied the images and made photographs in platinum prints. I used Bastian, David, and even French Chris for the photographs. Making the images was effortless because we had every object in the book from David's mad collecting. I asked Howard Read

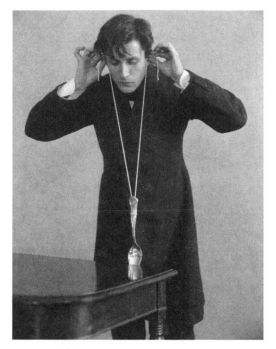

We took this picture of French Chris in *Les Récréations scientifiques*.

if maybe we could be included in the Biennial. Finally we were in, and we had a whole room to ourselves of twenty framed pictures with gold name placards attached describing each image.

John Patrick and Walter's house in the Catskills was split into apartments. They rented an upstairs one to a chubby woman who years before had approached David in Tompkins Square Park near Avenue A. We became friendly with her when we bought Oak Hill. She also lived around the corner from Avenue C. She was kind of fun but very self-absorbed and usually crying about some love affair gone wrong: a three-way, a current or former lesbian love affair, or some man that left after he went back to his wife. But I was very used to a narcissistic personality disorder.

Bastian and she got along and he'd take her on buggy rides. I did feel something was fishy, but since she was such a good friend I put my suspicions aside. But then Bastian started spending a lot of time in the country by himself. David threw an afternoon party at our country house one beautiful spring Sunday. Walter and John Patrick came, and we were going to take the train together back to the city. David mostly stayed upstate with Bastian to work on the property. This woman, whom I'll call Mallory, came to the party all dolled up in a dress, heels, and full makeup, along with four candle figures of three men and one woman from a voodoo shop. This seemed very odd but I didn't really think anything of it until I was on the train with John Patrick and Walter.

At the time McD, Bastian, and I were vegans. I was talking about the health benefits, as most vegans like to take over food conversations. John Patrick was looking a bit peeved at me. He then blurted out, "You're not *all* vegans!"

"What do you mean?" I asked.

"Well, some of you eat fish!"

I knew it wasn't McD or me.

"What do you think those fucking candles she brought to the party were for?" he said.

"What are you saying?"

"Nothing, Peter—I'm sorry I brought it up."

"Would you please just stop being so secretive and say what you mean!" Now I was upset. I tried to hide it because I knew he wouldn't tell me if I was upset, so I kept my suspicions to myself and tried to look calm.

"Okay, I'll tell you. Weeks ago, I was at the house to see Bastian and I went to the barn to find him and peeked in and saw him in a mount-down with her on a bale of hay!"

We were on a train back to New York much before the advent of cell phones. I felt trapped and livid as Patrick continued. "They all knew what was going on—all her little bitches knew, and I couldn't stand it any longer seeing them smile and side-eye each other at your party. I'm sorry, Peter. I really am." I was crushed right there. I had paid for Mallory to go on a meditation weekend to an ashram and was crying to her about how distant Bastian was being with both McD and myself. I had suspected something was wrong, but I didn't suspect this. I had lent her a full suite of Eastlake-designed furniture for her neighboring house, including a large eighteenth-century cabinet for dishes, and had helped her set it all up. I went back to Avenue C feeling like a huge fool. The next day I went to the studio while David and Bastian were still upstate and called Mallory's house. She answered and was happy to hear from me. My blood was boiling at this point. I tried to contain myself.

"How long have you been sleeping with Bastian?" I said coolly as I gripped the hard Bakelite receiver.

"Who told you?"

"Does that really matter now?" I snapped.

She stuttered.

"What the fuck were you thinking?" I screamed louder "I THOUGHT WE WERE FRIENDS, YOU FUCKING BITCH!" The rest of the conversation was more name-calling and screaming from me. I hung up the phone in the office of the studio.

Ten minutes later Bastian called, all chipper. "Hi, Peter—what's up?"

I knew she had run over to tell him, which annoyed me even more.

"What the fuck do you think is up, you little whore? I mean, really—you couldn't get someone better-looking or your own age?" I don't remember much else but more screaming from me. I hung up and was so relieved that this would be the end of him and he'd finally leave our house. I was thrilled to have him go. I wanted to get back to my life with David. I felt a sense of relief that I would no longer have to be with him and his distant, secretive behavior. Odd memories came up of different young woman "friends" who always seemed to be around. Soon the phone rang again.

"It's David."

I could tell he was with Bastian. Since we didn't have a phone upstate, these calls were all from a friend's house. I let out a tirade of fuming rants as my anger became demonic.

"Peter, you have to calm down. It's not good for you to be so upset."
I kept screaming.

"I'll call you later when you calm down."

In a couple of days, they came back home. I wouldn't talk to Bastian. But McD begged me not to throw him out. "I can't live without him!" he cried. I couldn't believe that he wasn't upset. Now I really felt completely alone.

David suggested that the three of us have a meeting at the studio. I sat far apart from them in the twenty-five-hundred-square-foot painting room. Bastian said he only had sex with Mallory once. Typical answer, I thought as I sat in silent contempt. So he stayed, saying he would never see her again. I had malicious contempt for him now. And his brother had been our bookkeeper whom we let go. There had been seven hundred dollars in our secretary's, Jane's, desk. The day he left, it went missing. Jane scoured her office for the money, tearing the writing desk apart. After many calls to him, he said he would be in the next day. He went to her desk and said, "Here it is," as he held up her cash payroll. Jane went over to it and said, "Thank you," as she grabbed it out of his hands.

16

Our friend Adrian Gilboe, who had a shop on East Tenth Street that we passed every day to and from our Brooklyn studio, was having a Halloween party at his run-down home in the Bronx. His little daughter was always dressed in Victorian black frocks, as though it were Halloween, and had a plastic skeleton as a doll. I wore a ragged nineteenth-century ginger-colored clown outfit with a pointed matching hat. Bastian fit into one of our original ladies' "suffragette" outfits. McD was mad at him and took off his bustled-dress outfit and refused to go.

The house was an old dump, beautifully appointed with antique furniture, but everything was threadbare and full of dust. No Halloween decorations were needed. They made an acid-green punch in a fish tank, and I was warned of its potency. I was soon to find out how haunted this house was. By the time the large fish tank was empty I wanted to leave but couldn't find Bastian. I went up the dirty wooden staircase and found our hostess, Thea, and her rock groupie friend, Cynthia, giggling outside a bedroom door. "What's so funny?" I asked.

"Oh, nothing!" The drunken women giggled some more. Now they were annoying me.

"Have you seen Bastian?" I asked. More giggling.

I heard some moaning from behind the bedroom door. I pushed it open to find Bastian with an old acquaintance I knew from her junk store in the East Village. They were in a heated embrace. In a rage I screamed at Bastian, "*What the fuck are you doing?!*"

The junk-store maven stood up. I saw Bastian's blank, drunken expression as behind me the women's giggling became laughter. I turned and screamed at them to go. The woman in the bedroom stumbled toward me, saying, "It's not what it looks like!" She wrapped her arms tightly around me, and I pushed her away. She flew across the room and landed on her back with her miniskirt covering her head, exposing her nudity.

I remembered a story McD told me of the junk-shop maven coming to his apartment on Avenue B for a party. She was dressed in a punk outfit with one breast exposed, safety pins, and her hair in turmoil. Nana was at that party and saw her and whispered to David, "Oh, that poor girl! I know what she's doing—but that's no way to get a man!" Well, she had a man now. I furiously went downstairs and told Adrian I wanted to leave and could he call a car service. Taxis, he told me, rarely ventured into his neighborhood. I understood as I peered out through the dirty lace curtains to a deserted street. I had to wait for a car. Thea and Cynthia came over to tell me everything was all right and not to get upset. I ignored them. Adrian had an old purse-sized gun he had been hoping to restore for Bastian. He handed it to me, saying he couldn't repair it. I put it in one of my large clown pockets.

Bastian stumbled down the stairs toward me. I didn't want to talk with him, but he wanted to. "Peter, I like women."

"Yeah, no kidding. What are you? The first closet heterosexual?"

The car came at around two a.m. and I left the house and jumped in, hoping to leave Bastian behind, but he ran after it and slid in next to me. After I told the driver the address in the East Village, I took the pistol from my pocket and threw it at Bastian. "Here's your stupid gun!" He threw it back at me and then I did the same till the driver stopped in the middle of a deserted Bronx highway and told us to get out.

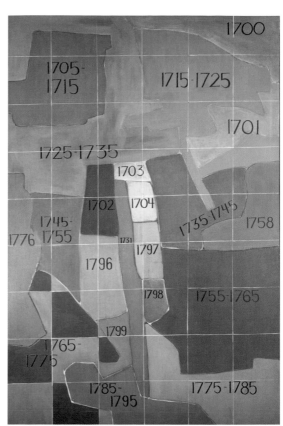

18th-Century Time Map, 1972, 1986
Oil on cotton, 108" x 72"

We made this in Pat Hearn's gallery
on Avenue B and Sixth Street for
Massimo's show about time.

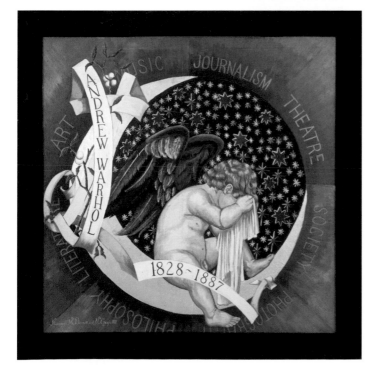

*Andy Warhol in
Memoriam, 1887, 1987*
Oil on linen, 70" x 70"

We did this painting
out of our admiration
for Andy Warhol.

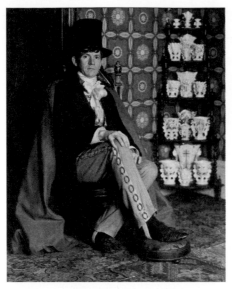

Portrait of the Artist with His Spill Vases, February 28, 1907, 1989 Cyanotype, 10" x 8"

A cyanotype print of McDermott on his thirty-seventh birthday in a copy of a nineteenth-century frock coat suit

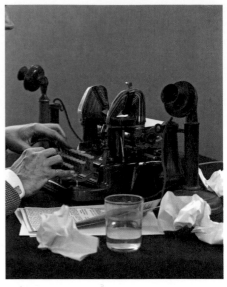

One of the First of Many Lovely New Printing Machines, November 17, 1895, 1989 Palladium print, 10" x 8"

A platinum-palladium print of one of our antique typewriters

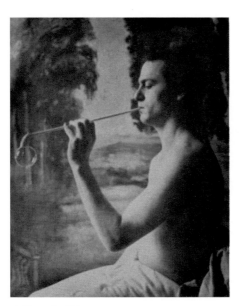

A Soap Bubble, 1915, 1989 Gum bichromate print, 30" x 24"

I learned by accident that during development, when this kind of print is submerged in water, the touch of a brush lifts the emulsion off, creating highlights.

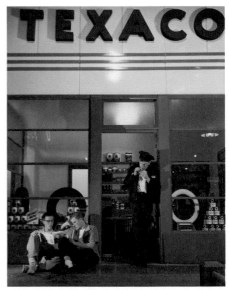

Cigarette Break, 1958, 2007 Carbro print 23 ¾" x 18"

A tri-colored carbro print from our portfolio *Detroit,* shot in the Henry Ford Museum

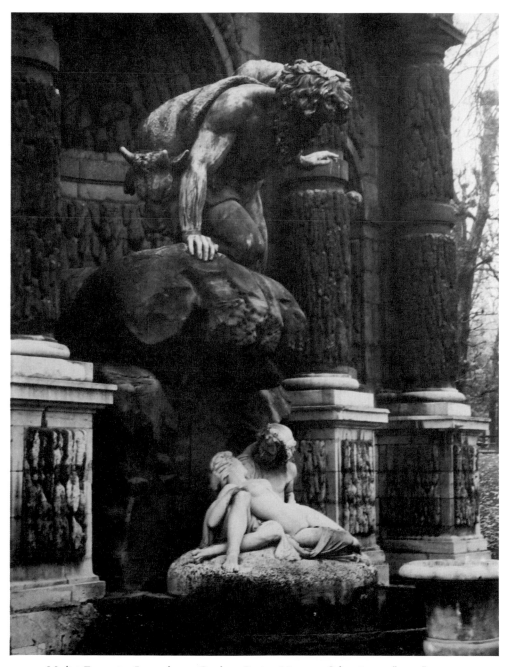

Medici Fountain, Luxembourg Gardens, Paris, 1865, 1994 Salt print, 24" x 20"

This salt print, made from a process invented in 1830 by Henry Fox Talbot, was part of a portfolio of French gardens commissioned by Harry Lunn, Jr.

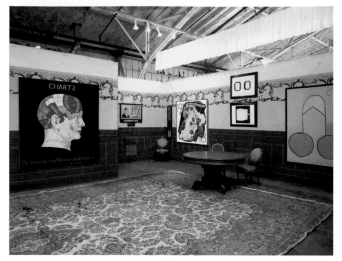

We painted the backdrops for our installation in the Sperone Westwater booth at the Chicago International Art Exposition, May, 1990.

Our show, *Velvet Rage, Flaming Youth, and the Gift of Desperation,* at the James Fuentes Gallery on Delancey Street in New York, 2015. The table was inspired by Catherine the Great's secret cabinet of erotic curiosities, which was destroyed during World War II. The urns are our version of erotic Greek pottery.

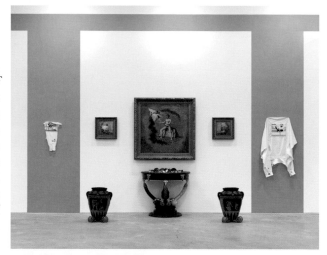

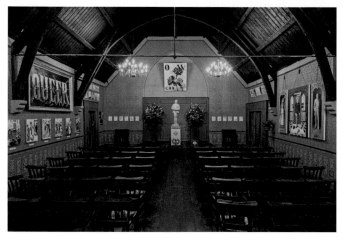

The Oscar Wilde Temple we created in Studio Voltaire, London, 2018–19. A contemporary space was converted into an Aesthetic Movement temple with wallpaper, stained-glass windows, nineteenth-century chandeliers, and a raised wooden floor.

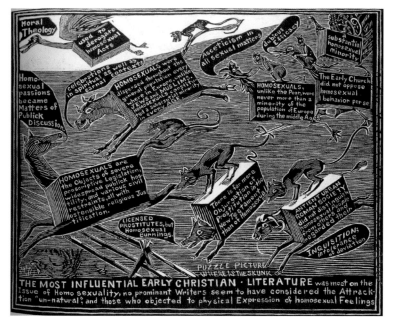

Conspiracy Painting IV, Homosexuality in the Middle Ages, 1928, 1997
Oil on linen 30" x 36"

These paintings, done in our studio in Dublin, were inspired by all the conspiracy books and articles McDermott read.

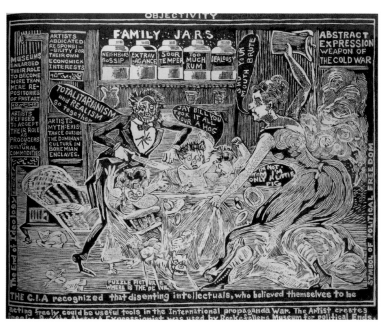

Conspiracy Painting VI, Abstract Expressionism: Weapon of the Cold War, 1928,
1997 Oil on linen 30" x 36"

This was influenced by a 1970s *Artforum* article.

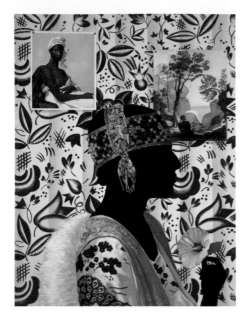

Portrait of Nancy, 1996
Oil on linen, 36" x 24"

In the 1980s, Bruno Bischofberger's clients commissioned many silhouette portraits; this was a portrait we made through the gallerist Jérôme de Noirmont.

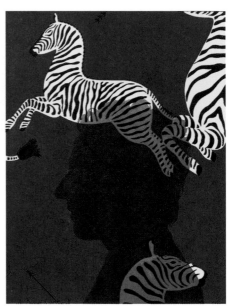

Portrait of a Designer, 2015
Oil on linen, 24" x 18"

This sitter wanted the Scalamandré wallpaper that had been in the iconic New York restaurant Gino's.

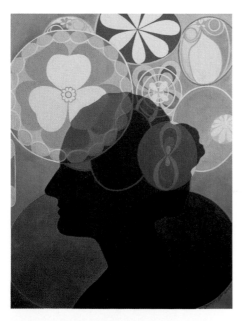

Portrait of a Lady, 2015
Oil on linen, 24" x 18"

This sitter asked to have the paintings of Hilma af Klint as her background.

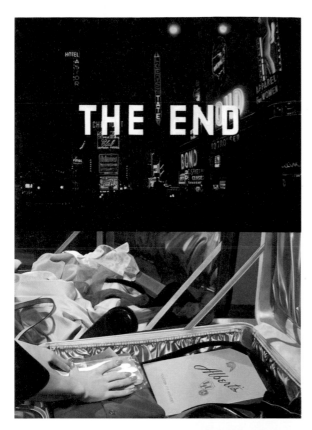

The Shadows Fall, 1966, 2008
Oil on linen, 84" x 60"

In 2005 we started our film-
still paintings, based on my
childhood obsession with old
movies and particularly with
that moment when the star
was suffering and making a
life-changing decision.

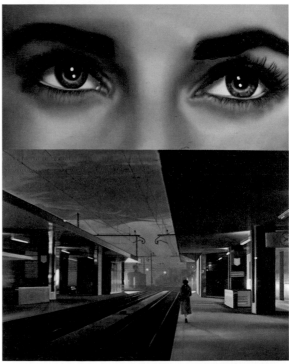

My Echo My Shadow, 1967,
2012 Oil on canvas, 60" x 40"

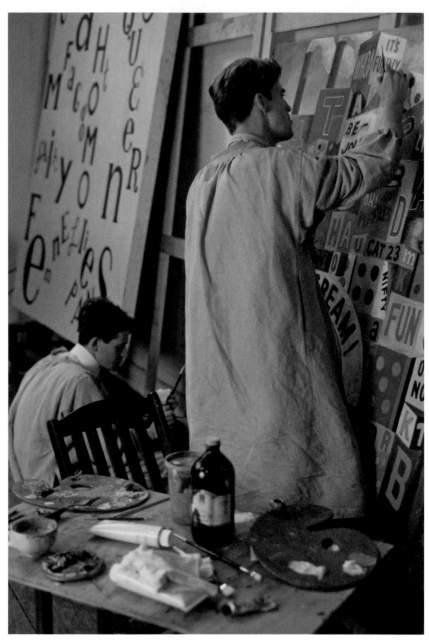

David and I are working on *It's a Scream,* 1987, at Julian Schnabel's studio, which he lent to us, at 77 White Street, above the old Mudd Club. It was included in that year's Whitney Biennial.

"I'm not getting out!" I screeched as Bastian opened the car door and threw up.

The driver came and opened my door and screamed, "Get out! *Get out!*" He pulled me out of the car, closed the back doors, and took off. I had no idea where I was, so I crossed the highway with Bastian following behind me. I was cursing him out for lying and using us for money. "If you're straight, what the fuck are you doing with two big fags? Huh? What are you, a gigolo?" I walked up a small hill as the car came back toward us. I was livid, ready to tell off the driver—till a cop car pulled up next to him.

"Those are the ones with a gun," the driver said to the cops, pointing at us.

"Whose gun is this?" they asked.

"His!" I raged, pointing to Bastian.

They immediately handcuffed him and started pushing him toward the backseat of the police car.

"Wait!" I screamed. "It doesn't work and there are no bullets!"

Realizing they didn't care, and not wanting to be left in the middle of nowhere on a cold highway, I asked if I could go along. We arrived at the station and they took Bastian into a cell as I waited for him on a wooden bench in the old police station which looked like something right out of a film noir. An hour later they brought Bastian out and he asked for his gun. The cop at the desk said, "This would be nice for my gun collection," and placed it in his desk drawer. McD warned me about the police so I very politely asked how we could get home and if they could call us a car.

"The subway's right there," he snapped, turning away.

We entered the empty station and waited about fifteen minutes for a train. Bastian threw up on the tracks. When an empty car stopped in front of us, I decided it would be safer to move to a car with people in it. As soon as the clown and the suffragette entered and sat down, we received a burst of laughter. I couldn't have cared less by now. It was nearly four a.m. We had to get off and change trains three times so Bastian could throw up again. Just before dawn we ended up home. I went into McD's room to get my stupid outfit off. I told him the story, saying that Bastian had to go, that he was just using us, liked women, and should live with someone he wanted to be with. I used a lot of profanity.

"You've got to calm down, Peter, and cursing's not going to help. Just go to bed and we'll talk about it in the morning." I felt sick the next morning, and Bastian was in a drunken coma. McD wasn't upset as long as he could hold on to his relationship with Bastian.

Bastian and I kept away from each other, and as I didn't have my former relationship with McD, I reinstated old friendships and courted new ones.

We were preparing a show for the larger space in the Miller Gallery for the beginning of 1992. The smaller space, where we first showed, went to Robert Graham, the classical sculptor. I started making large photographs with a difficult Victorian process called gum bichromate so that I could use watercolors in the printing process. I knew about a nineteenth-century German photographer, Heinrich Kühn, who used

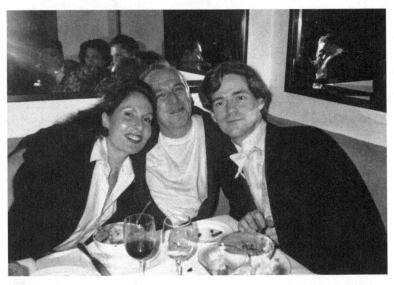

Jacqueline, Rene, and I at dinner after the opening of the Mammoth Photographs show at the Robert Miller Gallery, 1992

it beautifully in his images with only the color rust. But I thought it would be good to use many colors. I could take a brush while the image was underwater and remove the pigment to create the highlights. It looked like a beautiful monochromatic pastel. As it was nearly Christmas and McD and Bastian were heading upstate, I stayed in the city finishing the prints for the framers. I went up for Christmas Eve and returned the day after Christmas. The show was a success and got a half page in the *Times* with photos by McD's old friend Bill Cunningham of people who had come. A rude Lauren Bacall came with a lovely Anjelica Huston, who a few months later married Robert Graham. Later in 1992 another set of our prints traveled to the Fraenkel Gallery in San Francisco. Since we didn't fly, we took a train to Chicago and then on to LA to see Kristian on our way to San Francisco. Bradley had died of AIDS while living in a tent in Tompkins Square Park. The last time I saw Bradley he was standing outside the park on Avenue A crying loudly, "Someone please help me, I'm starving!" I went up to him: "Bradley, are you okay?" He immediately stopped crying and said, "Oh, yeah—ya knows, just working the corner trying to make a living." I gave him what I had in my pockets.

Bastian joined us in LA, as he had been in Virginia with Cowboy Bob, training horses. He now had a very different, distant attitude. One day we were sitting outside and he seemed particularly reserved, and then calmly stated that he wanted us to legally sign over one third of our estate to him. I could tell the Cowboy had his ear. It sounded just so legal and unemotional. "For what?" I said. "Driving cars, horses, and reading? You can forget it—ask one of your girlfriends."

Suddenly, McD chimed in. "You can have half of my half, Bastian."

I walked back into the house. It was a cold war between the pale Narcissus and me now. We were civil, and sometimes even chatty, but I never spent time with him alone. I worked making those shows, doing business, meeting deadlines, and I was not going to hand over one third to a layabout and now a practicing heterosexual.

We continued our train trip to San Francisco. At dinner we went into the dining car and asked for a vegetarian meal. They only had steak and potatoes with a salad. David politely asked if they could take the steaks off the plate, but said that we would still pay for them. The waiter kept refusing his repeated requests, so McD, in a rage, pushed our dinners off the table and went back to his seat in another car. Then the waiter came with the conductor and threatened to throw us off the train. Our demons were surfacing.

We arrived in San Francisco and had a crowded opening and good sales. On our return to New York, Angela Westwater asked us to come up with another idea for a solo show at the Park Avenue Armory art fair. We decided on paintings of furniture we saw in a 1908 Sears, Roebuck catalog. Angela gave us a check to get started. We bought all the canvases and stretched the linen and blocked them out. McD wanted to use a technique with thin lines that he started to lay down using skinny tape and painting in between with many colors to create a rippled effect over the furniture. But more fighting ensued. At this point I was angry most of the time—so angry that McD said to me, "I just wait for the time when you're not being a bitch, so I can have a nice conversation with you." I was in a bad mood most days. I was reclusive and miserable. After much angry badgering from me, McD went upstate with Bastian and said, "Finish them by yourself."

It was 1992, and the art market was beginning to feel the effect of Black Monday, so I let many assistants go. I had to finish the whole show with the taped lines David had begun, without him. The paintings were sent to the Armory. Only one small painting sold. We had never experienced that before. Angela and Gian Enzo were disappointed and sent the paintings back as soon as the Armory show ended. This was the first sign that the market had affected us. Uptown on Fifty-Seventh Street, Howard said, "It's a bloodbath out there." Now we were letting even more assistants go, then our chef. I let our British secretary, Jane, who was Jacqueline's former nanny, go. We needed money badly. I went uptown to the Miller Gallery to ask for help. Robert Miller was very cheery and walked me into his office while telling me he was part of the one percent. I had never heard that term before. As I sat down he asked, "Where are you going?" "I'm not leaving the gallery," I replied.

Amazingly—and I still can't believe I did it—I asked if he could give us two hundred and fifty thousand dollars. It didn't land well. I went back to the studio, to the dismay of McD. He wanted us to go back to see Miller, with Bastian. "Just wait for me—I want to finish this part of the painting," I said.

They didn't want to wait and went by themselves. I reminded him he could be risking utter ruin. Gone were our days of Divine Mind, when everything was "perfect." We had burned through millions over the years and owned nothing but Oak Hill. The cars and horses were in Bastian's name. I was too dumb to notice what he was doing.

It was a while before they came back from uptown, disappointed. What happened was that Miller wouldn't see him, and McD had started screaming in the gallery that he wanted money. Howard was out of town for all this. We mostly dealt with Howard since he sold the photographs. Howard called and asked me what had happened. I said I wasn't there, but we needed money. "Everybody needs money!" was his answer. Howard did incredibly well with our photographs. They were always on a shelf in the showroom, and he sold quantities of framed images.

Howard came to the studio to try and work things out. McD and Bastian took over the conversation. They were adamant that they receive a quarter of a million dollars. Howard said that at this time, with the market the way it was, it was ridiculous to ask for such a sum. He showed us the paperwork for how much he made for us, but his evidence was ignored. I felt this was Bastian pushing David. He still hated the art world and would criticize me for being stupid and weak. "Those merchants!" he'd taunt. Being alone with David was almost impossible. The few chances I had, McD wouldn't listen, so I just gave up. That was the last time I saw Howard as our dealer. We asked for the return of our photographs, but we owed the gallery thirty-three thousand dollars in framing costs. Julian helped us out and wrote a check. David went over to Julian's studio and gave him triple that amount in the returned photographs. Months later we ran into Howard near Sheridan Square, but he ignored us and kept on walking. Bastian asked why he didn't say hello. I flew into a rage, trying my best to maneuver my flurry of emotions, and said vehemently, "What do you expect him to say?" He feigned indifference. Then Sperone Westwater dropped us. But we still owed Gian Enzo a very large sum of money, too. Then the San Francisco gallery never spoke to us again. We were box-office poison.

Somehow, during all this we had agreed to let a young German woman named Barbara, who was at the NYU film school, make a documentary about us. Over the years, we had many people from all over the world wanting to photograph, videotape, or interview us, and McD was always very good with the press. Through our friend the filmmaker Emile de Antonio, he set up a meeting with a producer from *60 Minutes*. We lunched at a now defunct restaurant on East Seventh Street. The producer, along with de Antonio's wife, Nancy, and me, listened as David revealed his theories of time ("All time exists at the same time"), religion ("I want to start one"), sex ("Homosexuality is the norm, and it keeps population overgrowth down"), corporate America ("They own the government"), and more. We met De and Nancy the next Sunday for lunch, as we usually did, and asked about the *60 Minutes* producer. "Well," De explained, "he said that the viewers would think that David believes all of what he said."

"Of course I do!" David screeched. "So now no *60 Minutes* show? That's ridiculous!"

The day for the appointment with Barbara arrived. In walked a tall, beautiful blonde in her twenties. She was wearing a 1940s-style suit and had had the skirt made into hot pants to show off her long legs. I noticed Bastian's interest when he saw her. I asked her to pay us fifty dollars each for the days we shot. She reluctantly agreed since she was still a student. She had a somewhat big crew of other students and a professional cameraman. She had a story line to her film, not just questions. She'd film us painting upstairs, or using one of our large cameras making a picture in the sun-drenched studio. She used extras as our assistants, since by now we had fired them all. She had us act out her scenarios and let us change them if it worked. She filmed us in our Model T in Times Square and the horse and carriage in Brooklyn. Basically, we acted out our lives.

One day in the middle of shooting there was a knock at the side door. We were filming in our studio on the ground floor. It was three people from the IRS: two white men and a black woman in suits who ordered their way inside. "We've come to collect payment," one of the men said. They sat down right in the middle of the shoot at our large boardroom table with their McDonald's lunches and started eating while making jokes about us in a stage whisper. I told the film crew to go outside while I spoke with them. Since we didn't have any money, they took all of our framed photographs we had just received back from the Robert Miller Gallery. They took about $250,000 market-value worth of images. We had been called to their offices a month or so before and they had told us how much trouble we were in and how they would make us pay for ignoring them.

Howard called me and said that Sotheby's had all seventy photographs and were going to put them up at auction. Harry Lunn, who had started to represent us, called Sotheby's and bought them all for fifteen thousand dollars. When I asked to buy them from him he said, "No, these are mine." What could I do? He was our only dealer, and I didn't have any money. With the bad art market, the photos were cheaper and easier to sell now than paintings. Then Oak Hill was seized and locked by the IRS with orange stickers on all the doors and windows, including the general store.

We now were so paranoid we took our best furniture out of Avenue C and brought it to Jacqueline's house and left some paintings at Julian's studio. Jacqueline didn't like Bastian. She said he made David mean and critical. More than once she said to me, "You look so miserable." I was. My life was falling apart.

We were back to being poor again, with meager finances, but now owing so much money in back taxes and rents as well as our balloon payment of fifty thousand dollars due soon for Oak Hill. I felt like all my hard work had been for nothing. I hated Bastian—and then he started an affair with Barbara who was now my friend. He'd spend nights in her apartment. One evening in a fury I walked over to her building and shrieked up at the light in the casement, calling him a whore and a user as my voice echoed. No one answered or opened a window. I felt like a raging fool. I had no other outlet. I walked back home cursing myself for being such an idiot—not just for screaming up at a window but for the whole mess. The irony was that I was the one who had handed him the card back at the prep school. David seemed fine sharing him with her. At the same time as Barbara, Bastian was seeing a beautiful, rich young woman from India. He'd ask one out over the phone in the hall, and when the other woman was supposed to see him he'd come up with a lie. One day, a young woman who had been at the Egyptian fête came to the door asking for him. She had a wrapped present to give to him. I was in my bathrobe and slippers. I said in my best Bette Davis /Baby Jane Hudson voice, "He ain't here," and closed the door. How was I going to get him out of our lives? What mattered to me was my relationship with David and the art. Now I had this pile of property and no money to pay for it. I was walking with David and Bastian along Tompkins Square Park among the tents of homeless people and suggested that Bastian move in with Barbara, since he liked her so much. He grew enraged that I was trying to get rid of him. I played it nice to this arch-deceiver, saying I just wanted him to be happy.

Bastian was planning a trip upstate to visit his mother. David wanted to go with him, but Bastian kept trying to discourage him, though he finally relented. I guess David was trying to hold on to a relationship that had long been over. On returning, McD told me of Bastian's cold-ness toward him. I felt bad for David, but the trip changed his attitude toward his acolyte. McD had lost affection for him and finally, after six years, agreed to ask him to leave. He finally saw that what he was doing with these young women, he was doing with us. Walking home by myself one evening, I found an old ten-cent novel, *A Fool There Was,* on the street that was made into a silent movie with the vamp Theda

Bara. I picked up the book and took it with me. McD used to say the ancient Romans believed in signs from the gods. Was this my sign?

Bastian finally moved to Woodstock. McD took to his bed and wouldn't get out of it for weeks. He became completely despondent. He didn't talk much and ate his meals mostly in silence and would then go back to the big *baldacchino* bed and hunker down in the feather mattress. I had learned how to take care of things, but our situation now seemed out of control. With both of us depressed, I soon gave up. I put all the mail in a basket and ignored it. I didn't care anymore. Then the three-day auction in Albany of our belongings from Oak Hill came up. We weren't there when the trucks arrived to empty the house. The three cars, the horses, the custom tack, and all Bastian's belongings were already with him, since they were in his name and he had already moved out to his new place in Woodstock. I also gave him the portrait we painted of him in Capri and some photographs I took of him.

The auction date was announced, and Barbara said she'd drive us and help out. I went around with her to different bank machines as she took out six thousand dollars. We arrived three hours late, and people were busy bidding. The cinder-block warehouse in Albany was set up with a podium for the auctioneer and our belongings on either side. We found seats in the front and started bidding. We had contracted a lawyer before who said not to worry, he'd handle it. We later found out, from no returned calls, that he hadn't: he went on vacation for a month without telling us, and then it was too late. I saw a plump, dark-haired woman in glasses and a messy ponytail with our tailor-made eighteenth-century *incroyable* clothing of knee britches, waistcoats, and numerous scarves made in different colored silks. We had them made for a baroque ball in Vienna that we ended up not going to. I begged to buy them back. She replied, "No way—my friends and I like to get dressed up and ride horses." I followed her and begged her to give me my father's First Communion picture, which she held in her hand. She let out a big, annoyed sigh and handed it back to me and turned away.

Justin showed up carrying his paper bag, his coffee, and his long cigarette and lamenting our fall and commenting on each piece held up by assistants. He sat in the front row with us. "This is outrageous!" he screeched, turning to the crowd and making loud comments on how horrible the antiques dealers were to be trying to buy it all back. There on folding chairs sat all the dealers we knew and had supported. I went to greet them and asked them to please let me buy our things back. "Yes, yes," they'd say, and then bid against me as I walked back to my seat. They said little to me and continued buying. McD went outside as I bid on some things. The Warhol eighteenth-century bench came up, and it went higher than I could afford. Each piece had a story and a memory for me: the nineteenth-century crystal champagne flute we bought in Naples, or a beautiful eighteenth-century wooden chair I meticulously scraped decades of paint off for weeks, making a mixture of all the different colors blending underneath in powdery shades of green and pink. During a break I went up to the auctioneer and said that selling mattresses and flags was illegal, so he let me take our foot-high feather mattresses and nineteenth-century flags and put them in our pile of things. Then I went outside to find David. He was sitting on the parking lot macadam in his white suit with his head bowed down and his boater hat covering his face. He was sitting in the dirt against a chain-link fence matted with weeds. I was shocked to see him sitting in the muck.

"David," I begged, "get up, you're sitting in the dirt."

"I just can't believe this is all happening." The scorching sun above had lit up the parking lot, and his white clothes were blinding me.

"I know, it's horrible. But don't sit there—you're ruining your suit."

"I don't care. I don't care about anything. Why should I bother—for what? It's all gone, anyway. Everything's ruined."

I helped him up and brushed the back of his clothes and brought him inside. His mood was like that of a patient after a lobotomy. He was a dead man walking. Justin and Barbara were still inside in the front row. I sat bidding, zombie-like, not speaking with them. McD would come in, stay a bit, and go back outside to sit by the chain-link fence. At the end of the last day we packed up the belongings we had bought back with the six thousand dollars from Barbara. I looked over the room and saw an Empire sofa that we had used in our photographs. The move had broken its already delicate frame. I left it where it sat.

After the first day of the auction Justin had invited us to his new place in Albany. It was in a terribly run-down neighborhood. We were shocked by the house he was living in, which was on its last legs. This made any slum we lived in look like a palace. He had the street-floor apartment down a side street. The low wattage of the lamps kept it quite dim. But as usual he made a certain sissy magic out of scraps. It had all his usual trappings of wax-covered candlesticks and shredded upholstered sofas and chairs covered in bits of fabric. A ratty old black lace veil covered a modern lampshade, and beautiful objects were mixed with his broken belongings. His bed was an Empire sleigh bed draped in bits of fabric to mock a *baldacchino*. And of course, a battered TV was on with no sound, and there was the same pink marble ashtray of cigarette butts. He gave us some tea and continued to lament the horror of the auction till David couldn't take it anymore and said we had to go.

We returned to the empty house in Oak Hill, where we slept on a mattress on the floor, using the old threadbare woolen flags as bedding. There was nothing else left except some unmarked tin cans in the little pantry. It was beyond depressing. We both stayed silent on how unhappy we felt. And then our balloon payment of fifty thousand dollars was due. We barely had fifty dollars. The owner who held the mortgage had told us earlier that he would refinance it for us, but he changed his mind. He took the property back, though we could stay there till the date of eviction.

The weeks after the auction are all a blur now. I had to pay Barbara the six thousand she loaned me, so I called a friend from Mexico and borrowed it to pay her back. I gave him some salt print photographs as remuneration.

17

With Bastian gone and in the aftermath of the auction, I was left trying to hold things together. All I could think was what a waste, with over a decade building a large life with David, not only the paintings and exhibitions but also our homes. Such attention had been paid to every little detail, and all it took was less than six months to have every bit of it slide off a cliff. The art market was collapsing, and there had been more than a decade of AIDS deaths.

One morning David came to my room. "I am going to move to Ireland," he said softly.

"What? Why do you want to go there?"

"There is nothing left for me here." His voice was uncommonly soft.

"You mean for good?"

"Yes. I want to leave as soon as possible."

"What am I supposed to do?" I cried out.

"You can come later."

"I don't want to move there," I said. "We don't know anyone there except Michael O'Donoghue. What about our life here? And we don't have the money for a ticket on the *QE2*."

"I'm going to ask Nana for the money. I've made up my mind. I just can't take it here. I don't need to live in New York anymore. I know every street and corner. I'm going to live in Ireland. Artists don't have to pay taxes there. I want to live in a place where they protect their artists. They destroyed not just our lives, but a great art experiment, and I can't put it back together now."

"So I'm supposed to handle all this mess?"

"You'll have to. I can't take it anymore." He left my room and went back to bed.

I didn't say anything else.

I was surprised when Nana sent him five thousand dollars. With part of the money he bought a one-way ticket on the *QE2* and saved enough to get him to Connemara, in the west of Ireland, to see Michael O'Donoghue and his wife, Cheryl. Since it was early summer, he packed a steamer trunk with his summer whites, suits, shirts, detachable collars, and ties, and a suitcase for his shoes. And a dirty canvas bag he packed with organic fruits. Another satchel held his books, sewing, and some stationery. He had so much luggage we had to hire a van to move it to the docks on the West Side Highway. A porter took the mound of bags in a cart as David and I followed him under an arch of balloons while a quartet with an accordion played pop songs. We said our goodbyes at the ramp that led to the ship.

"Go upstairs to the parking-lot roof and I'll come to the balustrade," David suggested.

I went up to the roof and waited till he appeared. He came out and we spoke loudly to each other over the rail. Then a horn blew and soon the large vessel started to move backwards from the dock into the Hudson River. I walked to the end of the rooftop as the ship moved along, speaking with David. Then the ship turned and slowly sailed down Manhattan. David pulled out his handkerchief to wave goodbye, and I did the same until he became a small dot among many others. I turned and went down an escalator to the street and crossed the highway.

"He'll be back," I said to comfort myself. "He'll be back in less than a year."

I passed by where they kept the horse and carriages for Central Park. A cloud of depression engulfed me. I went to a run-down park, sat on a bench, and sobbed. I blamed myself for being a fool and a coward. If only I had had more belief in myself and had fought to keep it all going, but I couldn't or didn't. I had never before felt so lonely as I did on that sad little bench.

With John Patrick's help I sold the bank's office furniture and some other pieces from the studio, since no one was buying art from us. The new owner of Avenue C took me to court to pay the seven months of rent I owed. I lost the case. Then he sold the building to some gays and I was given a month or two to move. Meanwhile David was in Ireland, and I'd call now and then or get a collect call from him. He'd ask for some money. I tried to send as much as I could. Cheryl came to him one day and asked how long he'd be staying there. He didn't have an answer, so he knew he had to leave. They found him a "tigh," a little open shack with broken windows and no doors in a field where cows would enter and walk among the debris of old clothes and garbage inside. It had a little stair that went up to a small bedroom and the tiniest fireplace, no bigger than a portable TV. David fixed it up and repaired the door. One day he called to tell me about his life in the tigh. An elderly man came by to visit him. McD invited the man in and sat him by the fire. The man asked him if he was alone. David replied that he was. "I'm alone, too," the man said. "I take care of my mother. All my siblings have moved on except me." David nodded. Then the old man asked, "Since you're alone and I'm alone, do you think we could get together?" he asked suggestively. David told me he looked at the withered old man and thought, "Well . . . if I have sex with him, maybe some cute young fellow will want me the way he wants me."

"So," he told me over the phone, "I opened my sailor trousers and let the flap expose myself to him. Then the fellow jumped up and screamed, 'You're a man!'

"Well, I didn't know what to say," David continued, "so I buttoned my trousers up and the man became enraged and picked up the fire poker and started chasing me with it!"

I couldn't believe the story, and I burst out laughing. We hadn't laughed together like that in so long.

"Then on Sunday," David continued, "I went to church and sat in the front row. The rest of the elderly parishioners sat five rows behind me. No one would speak to me after the service." The locals had heard the story that he was having women in his tigh after he let a female hiker stay in a tent on the land. And the old seducer also wanted David out. Even the O'Donoghues thought he'd be better off in Dublin.

Now I had to pack up Avenue C. And our studio—the top floor of the bank—already had three floors of our belongings, including the stage from the Egyptian fête. So not only did I have to move out of the studio but also out of the house in Manhattan. Both properties were chock full of furniture, our costumes and extensive wardrobe of antique clothing, numerous objects, large wooden cameras, all the photos and their large negatives, plus our paintings and so much more.

For the next few months it was a daily trial of packing all the effects of our life. I found a company to move all the belongings and I could pay them later. I called some neighbors up in Oak Hill who had let us store things of ours in their barn. When I called to retrieve them, they told me they wanted a five-thousand-dollar storage fee. I was so shocked that I called John Patrick for advice. "I'll handle it," he said. He drove up to the mountains and threatened the people that if they didn't give back our belongings they'd have him to deal with. He succeeded in getting them returned.

I had a week left to get out of Oak Hill. My friend Paul Meleschnig drove me upstate to collect the few things I bought at the auction and our feather mattresses and flags. After we filled the car I said, "I just want to go back inside." It was my favorite property, and I wanted to see it one last time. I went into the house and looked through the empty rooms, from the parlor with its 1900 wallpaper, up the small mahogany-railed stairway with the original pink walls to the two bedrooms and dressing rooms. Bastian had the one with a columned fireplace. My room had the original paint on the wooden closet door. I closed all the shutters in both rooms. I went back downstairs and bolted the front door and placed the large brass key on a hook. I walked through the dining room into the kitchen, where we made our meals on a hook over the fireplace as we had done at Wardle House. I went up the worn stairs to where David slept. I just looked at the room and remembered bits of our happy conversations when we had first bought the house. I closed his bedroom door, went down the stairs, and walked out through the small pantry and placed the tiny lock on the back door, hiding the key under a rock as we had done so many times.

I went through the general store in all its stained-walled darkness and looked out the shop's windows which I used to decorate for the holidays. I went upstairs to the apartment, closed every door, and headed to the barns in the back where we had the carriages and to the paddock where the horses were kept. The homemade fence was still up. I passed the stone wall we paid fifty thousand for, to the stone steps to the creek we used to swim in. Again, I started to sob. I had spent very little time here since I was always working. Working for what, now? I walked back to the car. I took my seat next to Paul and said, "Let's get out of here."

I had finished packing the boxes from the two floors of Avenue C and then headed to tackle the Williamsburg studio. I rolled up our twenty-two-foot painting *Opium Smokers Dream* that we copied from a photo Michael Burlingham had of a painting belonging to his great-grandfather, Louis Comfort Tiffany, and put it with everything else going to Ireland. It was all taken and put in containers and shipped to the docks of Dublin. It was 1995, and with no place to live or work, I booked a flight to Dublin to live with David, who had rented a small house near Ballsbridge. We then started painting in the parlor floor, and after a while we rented a small art studio in Temple Bar in downtown Dublin on the River Liffey and were back again making art together and exhibiting. Bruno Bischofberger had many silhouette commissions for us, and through his ex-gallery director Andrea Caratsch we started showing with Jérôme de Noirmont in Paris. So, life was working on a much smaller scale, but after everything we went through I felt fine with it, even if I still missed our life and our friends in New York.

And then I didn't feel so well.

18

In my new town of Dublin, in the autumn of 1995, I went to have a
massage at a young woman's small house. As she was massaging me
she pinched my left big toe and I let out a scream. Later in the day my
foot slowly turned purple. Then, the next day, my leg started to swell
and ended up looking like a long purple balloon.

David took me to the hospital where I sat for two hours waiting to
see a doctor. After examining me they put me in the leg ward with an
antibiotic drip for a week. I was in the ward with six other men, separated only by a flowered curtain. McD brought me vegetarian meals
with juices each day, arriving in his winter cape and top hat.

After a week my leg swelling subsided and I went home. I went back
to painting, but my toe was still swollen and purple, and another spot
appeared on my ankle.

We had our studio and continued making work for European dealers. Our main dealer was Bruno Bischofberger, and through him we
met Prince Ernst August of Hanover, who wanted to commission silhouette portraits of his family. In the press he was known to be a wild
child, but to us he was very courtly. He also asked us to do his friend
Karl Lagerfeld's silhouette, which was to be a gift from him, and so I

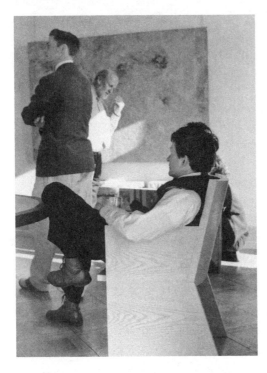

Visiting Bruno Bischofberger, center, at his gallery in Zurich. I am standing, McD is sitting.

arranged to fly from Dublin to Paris with the necessary paper, pencils, and candle.

When I arrived at Lagerfeld's house and atelier on rue de l'Université, he was not in, and an assistant had me wait in a room while his employees sat around gossiping, smoking cigarettes, and ignoring me. Then the Master walked in, and they all stood up, suddenly looking very busy. He couldn't have been more attentive to me and asked if I had been served lunch. When I said no, he loudly ordered them in French to get me a plate. Soon the group's mood toward me changed.

Lagerfeld apologized, saying that he had a bit of work to attend to. He sat down at a large round table as a group of seamstresses in white coats with wristbands of needles seemed to appear from nowhere. He dashed off a number of sketches of a dress on a large pad, ripped the sheets of paper off, and handed them to his seamstresses, who swiftly departed through the double doors. Next he had a hairdresser and a makeup artist come in. He drew how he wanted the hair and then the makeup, ripped those pages off, and quickly handed them over as they, too, left through the double doors. Finally we were alone, and since I had finished my meal, he said, "Shall we begin?" as he escorted me up a grand eighteenth-century staircase into a suite of white-and-gold-paneled rooms. I set my candle on a beautiful carved transitional table and lit the wax taper. He became very excited in the darkness with his shadow on the wall and asked his butler to get a camera. After I explained that the flash would destroy the shadow, he sent the man away.

I had complimented Lagerfeld on his high starched collar, a version of which McD and I always wore. He left the room and returned with a big blue box with one of his tailored shirts and a large black silk cravat and handed it to me. I was thrilled and thanked him for it. He then asked me if I would like a tour of his house, and he led the way, cooling himself with a white fan. Each room was more beautiful than the last, with statues, paintings, furniture, and porcelain. I felt like such a hick because all I could say was "oh" and "wow" as he pointed to objects. We continued past a small group of early-nineteenth-century portraits of men and women with elaborate coiffures and dress. In the next room I spotted a small papier-mâché centerpiece of trellises and flowers on a long table. Inside sat six small glass candlesticks. It somehow caught my attention and I asked about it. He sat across from me and said, "Thank you. This is very rare. These were used as centerpieces at parties and then usually thrown out. We found this one in an attic, where it had been left for over two centuries." It was soon evening, and we went into his garden which was a manicured square lawn surrounded by a gravel path with a leafless crooked tree right out of a symbolist painting. Even though it was chilly outside, he kept fanning himself. Full of awe, I said to him, "My goodness, you live in a dream!" He stood there in the moonlight and repeated in his deep French accent, "Yes, I live in a dream."

Ingrid Sischy, the former editor of *Artforum* and then *Interview* magazine, was a major supporter of our work. She was also a great friend of Julian's. She put us on the cover of *Artforum* in 1986 and hired me to shoot for *Interview*. I had called her up at the office and asked if I could interview the top gay porn star of the moment, Jeff Stryker. In the old world of porn he was the most famous, so famous they made a dildo of his penis. Ingrid often invited McD and me to small lunches or parties at the *Interview* offices with people who had been featured in the magazine.

One day in 1996, she called me up and said she had spoken to Elton John and Gianni Versace about our work and wanted to bring them to the studio. But it turned out that neither of them could make it to our Williamsburg studio. At the time, people couldn't believe we moved our studio so far away. "It's only one stop in Brooklyn on the train," I would emphasize to try to get them there. Instead, Ingrid arranged for me to go visit Versace at his town house uptown. On the appointed day, just as I walked through the door, he appeared to welcome me with his boyfriend, Antonio D'Amico. "Please, please come in," he said.

A maid in a perfect uniform that looked as if she pressed it hourly served coffee and cakes on Versace china. After the cakes, Versace brought out a recent catalogue for a show of ours in Milan. He spoke with a high voice and in the third person. "What Versace is about is a-fashion, a-sex, and a-rock and roll," he said, rolling his *r*'s. "And everything he touches brings this out." He paused a lot as his Italian accent came through heavily.

He opened the pages of the catalogue and showed me a painting we did on an old backdrop from our booth at Sperone Westwater in Chicago. On it we painted a patented pattern of Y-front men's cotton briefs underwear from 1936, which later became sexualized and known as "tighty whities." He took the book and put it up close to my face. "Versace want this painting, but of course using Versace underwear"—the kind with a Medusa head on the waistband. "But Versace want the underwear to have a bulge." I went on to explain that it couldn't have a bulge because it was a sewing pattern.

"Versace want a bulge," he insisted, staring at me intently.

I was led by the two Italians to a large dressing room covered in mirrors. Versace then opened a long mirrored door, behind which there were towers of shelves with a multitude of different kinds of Versace underwear. He handed me a pair of black lace stretch boxer briefs (also available in white), see-through briefs of both colors with no lace, and then a pair of baggy soft-cotton boxers and the tiniest bikini-style underwear with a waistband that seemed bigger than the "panties." He started to hand me piles of different kinds in their store packaging. Antonio brought out a Versace shopping bag and dumped them all in.

He ended up ordering a few other versions of paintings from the catalogue and then gave me a tour of his house. We climbed a huge marble staircase, passing through the large marble foyer upstairs to a sitting room with Versace home furnishings and paintings by friends from the East Village: George Condo, Philip Taaffe, Schnabel, Warhol, and other luminaries.

A week later, he wanted to commission seven full-figured, life-sized silhouette portraits of his family members. I went back to the town house and this time his whole family was in an upstairs sitting room. We moved to a smallish, dark bedroom, and I set up a candle and began tracing their silhouettes: I drew Donatella; her husband, Paul Beck, and their children; Gianni's brother, Santo; and Antonio. Versace's nephew liked sneakers, had a large collection of them, and wanted to have his silhouette with his sneakers in color. Again I tried to explain that our work had historical references and that we backdated the artwork to suit the image. "Versace wants his nephew's portrait to have sneakers," was all he said.

Then he invited me to an Oscar party at the town house the following week. What does one wear to a Versace Oscar party? I wore an eighteenth-century ruffled shirt and a frock coat. I arrived the evening of the party, and as I got out of the taxi I saw a group of photographers who turned in unison at my arrival and started snapping. Then when they asked who I was, and learned I wasn't a celebrity, they lost interest.

A man in uniform let me in. I stood at the top of a small staircase as my host came to greet me.

"Ahhhhhh, looook!" said Versace, laughing. "It's Draaaaaacula!"

He brought me to meet the other guests. Molly Ringwald was there, and Philip Taaffe and his wife, Gretchen. We sat in front of one of the first huge flat-screen TVs, on which we watched the red-carpet appearances. Mira Sorvino was on the red carpet, up for Best Supporting Actress in Woody Allen's *Mighty Aphrodite*. "Oh, look at her!" Versace said. "It must be Armani's housewife clothes." He'd point out the celebrities who wore his own clothes. "Oh, yes, another beauuuutiful Versace dress!" he'd say, praising Versace's brilliance. "So beauuuuutiful!"

Soon after the Oscars began, Woody Allen showed up with Soon-Yi

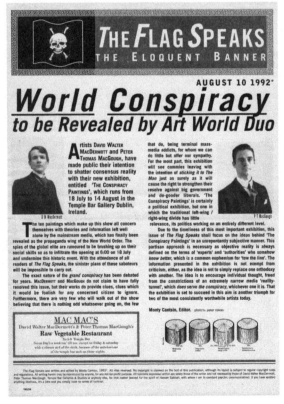

This was the catalogue for the *Conspiracy Paintings* show in Dublin.

Previn. Allen was one of McD's and my favorite directors, especially for *The Purple Rose of Cairo.* All I could manage to say was "Hello." He sat with Molly Ringwald and Philip Taaffe. I was awestruck and remained silent. I had seen all of his films. Then the time came when the Best Supporting Actress was announced, and Mira Sorvino won. Woody said how happy he was she won and how beautiful she looked. "Ahhh, yes," Versace chimed in. "Doesn't she look beautiful!"

I had made the silhouette deal with Versace, and he wanted to commission nine paintings. It was a big sale, and I felt proud of myself. But when I called Bruno in Zurich, he said the price was too cheap.

Later, when I was in Basel for the art fair, I ran into Ingrid. "How did it go with Gianni?" she inquired.

"Bruno doesn't want to do the deal. He says it's not enough. He should pay double," I replied.

"*What?*" Ingrid said. "Let's go see him now!"

I was filled with dread, imagining what would happen when these two powerhouses started talking. We found Bruno in his booth at the fair. Ingrid started asking him why he was canceling the Versace offer. Bruno answered in his deep, firm voice, "It's much too cheap."

The next thing I knew Ingrid left in a huff.

The following year, 1997, David and I were in Dublin preparing a show in the gallery below the Temple Bar studio of a group of nine paintings we called *The Conspiracy Paintings,* based on all the conspiracy books and articles David had read. Later those paintings went to a group show at Whitechapel in London called *Protest and Survive,* which Matthew Higgs curated.

So we were doing all right and had a studio manager and an assistant. One night I went to a U2 concert in an outdoor stadium with friends of the band. It wasn't cold out, but I was freezing. I was so cold I asked my friend Isabel for her large scarf to wrap myself in as I shivered. A week later I left for New York, and on the plane I found the air conditioning much too cold and asked that it be turned down, but I was still cold and ended up with four blankets covering my body from head to toe. Everyone else on the plane was fine.

In New York I saw Patrick and he gave me the number of his Park Avenue doctor. I wanted to know why my big toe was still purple. I sat in the waiting room with Upper East Side–looking women. The doctor was nice enough, and I showed him my foot and some more spots.

"Have you ever had an AIDS test?" he asked.

"No, I never did."

"Well, let's just try and see. Better to know."

My mind was racing. "Oh, no!" I thought. I didn't want to know, as the nurse stuck a needle in me while the doctor was finishing up.

"Call in two weeks and we'll give you the results," the receptionist said, as I paid in cash and took the doctor's card. Those two weeks were the longest two I've ever experienced. Images of my dying friends haunted my sleep. And then another purple spot appeared.

The time came to make the call. I entered an old glass phone booth uptown and dialed the number. Finally, the doctor came on the phone.

"Peter," he said dryly, "I don't have the news you're looking for. You tested positive for AIDS." The booth was suddenly silent, even with the noise of the traffic outside. I could hear my heart beating in my ears. I felt I was falling into an abyss.

My hand hurt from the strong hold I had on the phone. I softened my grip and listened.

"Are you still there?" the doctor asked.

"Yes," I whispered.

"You'll need to see an AIDS specialist," he continued.

I tried to listen, but I started to sob and hung up the phone mid-sentence. I put my head in the corner of the glass booth and wept. A knock at the folding door startled me. As I exited, uncontrollably sobbing, the woman apologized. Others waiting for a bus turned to stare at me, and I quickly turned and ran down the street. I turned up my collar and crushed my hat down below my brow to hide my face.

I was stunned, but what had I been thinking? I had seen so many men with purple spots on their faces, legs, and arms, and ones with sunken faces with skinny arms, bloated stomachs, and large swellings of fat in the back of their necks. All I could think of was the sickness and agony that awaited me. I looked at the multitudes of people on the crowded rush-hour streets and wished I could trade bodies with any of them.

Getting back to Jacqueline's, where I was staying, was a blur. I finally arrived, and luckily no one was home. I called a friend and told him, sobbing, how my life was ruined but begged, "Please don't tell anyone." I felt terribly alone in Jacqueline's big, empty town house. I climbed the creaky wooden stairs to my little room off the hall, closed the door, and cried myself to sleep.

I awoke in darkness and tried to go back to sleep, but soon it was morning, and I waited for the house to come awake. I went downstairs and saw Jacqueline having coffee. She has always had this funny way of knowing things I didn't want her to know. She asked if I was okay. After telling her I was all right, I told her I had to cut my visit short and return to Dublin.

Back in Ireland, after I told David, he recommended Christian Science and a raw-food diet. He had rented a large nineteenth-century house in the Swiss style, thirty minutes away from Dublin. The house had not been changed since 1905. Thieves had stolen the green marble and pink marble fireplace mantels from the parlor and the dining room. The furniture we had shipped over from Manhattan was still in storage because we didn't have the funds to get it out, and so David had moved into an almost empty house. The year we were there the house was robbed eight times. And it was another freezing house, with the only working fireplaces upstairs where the bath didn't work.

The kitchen, however, had a massive wood-burning stove to cook on and a hand pump for water that still worked. Since you couldn't unlock the house from the outside, when we wanted to enter we'd get a ladder from the barn and place it at an upper window, where we entered, and then go downstairs to unlock the kitchen door from the inside, then go back outside to put the ladder back, and then go back inside again. Leaving the house, we had to do it all over in reverse.

After a while I just couldn't eat. I had no appetite and only drank the fresh-squeezed orange juice McD's manservant, George, would make for me. He'd arrive with a knock on my bedroom door wearing his uniform, a Chinese opera costume with a cap that had a rope braid down the back. I'd drink the pint of orange juice (McD would collect the glasses off the streets of Temple Bar after the clubs closed) and stay in bed with the fire burning through the whole day into evening. I was so depressed I would just sit in a chair rocking and looking out my window to the forest across the lawn. One morning I spotted a sweet little squirrel eating a walnut that fell from a tree. This gave me such comfort—how beautiful nature was! Then a large gray rat came out of the brambles and attacked the squirrel and took the walnut. Somehow this set me off. I lowered my head and rocked, moaning, in the chair. I had given up. I didn't care anymore. I hated that house and I hated not being around my friends. And I was dying just like my friends did.

The spots started climbing up my leg to my stomach, chest, and then my face. I was covered in purple KS sores. Behind my ears they were like purple grapes. My foot would swell and ache, making it hard to even walk. But I sat there with no medication, believing that I would be healed by food. I knew my friend Tina Chow had died from no medication and a macrobiotic diet; we had gone to her funeral before McD left for Ireland. And Walter had an ex-boyfriend, a wine merchant, who died the same way, saying he was going to be cured by a healthy diet. Ignoring their example, I stubbornly persevered and stayed my course with juice and raw food. But all the chewing hurt my jaw, and the salads were too harsh on my stomach. My few friends in Dublin were horrified by my appearance.

I would go back and forth to New York, attending meetings for raw-food advocates in the back of a vegan restaurant. Some people were trying it to cure a disease and some just because they believed it was the way to eat. We sat in a circle on folding chairs and people spoke of their eating habits. One skeletal woman with a very skinny red braid she would fondle as she spoke was "mono eating," saying she only ate oranges. People would lament that they had "slips" and had eaten a pizza. The two who ran the meeting looked very healthy. One man was a lecturer on the benefits of raw diets, and I worked with him for a bit. I would go to his Upper West Side apartment and he would try to get me to exercise. I could barely do three push-ups before I needed to lie down on his sofa. He had a large table piled with the fruits and vegetables that made up his diet and presumably gave him his lean, muscular figure. He had no body fat and said that he knew what proteins and vitamins were in all foods.

He said I'd been ruining my body with a bad diet and drugs. I told him I hardly took any drugs, illegal or legal. I then met a young, muscular "breatharian," who claimed he survived on air alone. Surviving on New York City air? He couldn't meet me in his apartment, so we met in a retro diner on Avenue A. He took my pulse and scribbled notes on a piece of paper as I paid him the two-hundred-dollar fee in cash.

I felt grifted, but I kept going on eating raw food. I was invited to a dinner at Anna Wintour's house for an English artist and sat there eating only carrot sticks and celery, to the horror of those around me. I was as weak and thin as could be, and the purple spots kept coming. McD continued pushing raw foods, as did some of my friends.

When I was back in Dublin, the phone rang and it was Jacqueline. I was very happy to hear from her and get some relief from my anxiety. "I was wondering how you're doing," she said. I knew she knew. She had that sixth sense about her. I started to whimper as I told her what was happening. "I'm sick—I'm really sick. I don't know what to do."

"Look," she said, "we don't have to talk about it if you don't want to."

"No, I want to. I'm so tired of this sick secret!"

She listened to me as I slowly stopped crying and told her my story of visiting the doctor in Manhattan. I don't remember much more of the conversation, but ten minutes after I hung up the phone rang again, and it was Julian.

"Hi, Pete, it's Julian. Jackie just called me."

The tears flowed again, even more.

"Okay, Pete, now stop crying."

"I'm not going to stop!" I snapped back.

"Okay, okay, you don't have to stop. Now listen—get on a plane and come to New York. You can stay with me or Jackie."

"I can't come—I have to finish a painting commission and bring it to Bruno in Zurich. I need the money."

"Fuck the painting, man. Get to New York. I'll give you money."

"Stop, Julian—you're getting me upset."

Julian called about five times in the next thirty minutes.

"Hi, Pete—I called Ingrid and she's friends with Jerome Groopman, who's the top AIDS specialist in the world. He says there's a new drug they just came up with and people are living."

But I kept insisting on going to Zurich and getting the much-needed money. I left on a small plane Bruno's client sent and brought the painting to Zurich. I told people I was on a diet when they asked why I was so thin. I took the check and went to get a fresh juice in town. Oddly, I ran into Josef Astor, who had photographed David since the early seventies and took our picture for many magazines in the eighties. I saw the look of horror on his face. The spots were still visible through the heavy pancake makeup.

"Are you all right?" he asked. I joked off his concern and said I was fine.

I was also reading *The Cure for HIV and AIDS* by Dr. Hulda Clark, who had an office in Tijuana, Mexico, because the United States Trade Commission forbade her to practice in America. I went back to Ireland and got another call from Jacqueline. I agreed to leave Ireland, against the wishes of a very upset David, who did not want me going on the new drug. "Those drugs killed our friends, and I don't want you to die!"

"They said it was a new drug, not just AZT," I argued. "And I'm going tomorrow. Just look at me—I'm not getting any better."

Back in New York, when I arrived at Jacqueline's house she gave me a big hug. For such a glamorous, chic person she has the biggest heart of gold.

"I've bought two tickets to Boston to see Dr. Groopman. We leave tomorrow."

We took a morning flight and arrived in the doctor's office. Later Dr. Groopman came out and invited me into the examination room.

"Can my friend come with me?" I asked.

"I can wait here," Jacqueline said.

"Please, I'd like you to be with me."

I went behind a screen and undressed, then lay down on an examining table. I didn't have any makeup on that day. Dr. Groopman then began the exam. He looked over my front and back.

"Well, you certainly have many spots. I want to do an X-ray to see if you have them on your internal organs." He was very kind and gentle. I think he was used to his patients' fears.

After I dressed he sat me down and wrote three prescriptions. "Here, this is new, and it will help you. We've had a lot of success with the new drugs." He handed me the three pieces of paper.

My mood suddenly changed. "I'm not going to take this! This is what killed my friends!" I said hysterically.

He didn't even blink at my outcry. "I understand your fear. It's a new drug that we've had a lot of success with. Just take the prescriptions with you and see later what you think."

I took the prescriptions and said my goodbyes. I felt bad about my outburst because he was so kind.

Waiting for the plane back to New York, I talked to Jacqueline and she encouraged me to get the meds. I was suddenly feeling hungry and bought a large pretzel at a kiosk in the airport. It was the first cooked food I had had in months. I later threw it up in the toilet on the plane.

Back at her house, over morning coffee the next day, Jacqueline said she needed to talk. "Peter, you can stay here as long as you want. It doesn't bother me." She later told me she was considering hiring a nurse to take care of me. I was rail thin and covered in spots, and my clothes hung loosely on me. I was like a ghoul hanging around her house eating lettuce. Her kids were really sweet to me. The loveliest gift I ever received was from her daughter Lola, who gave me a bottle of the thickest makeup base they made wrapped in a beautiful red silk scarf. (I wore many scarves to hide my skinny neck and sores.) And Jacqueline kept telling me stories of friends who were being healed on the new pills. "You have to take them. I can't watch you die in front of us. It's too much and just too sad."

I agreed and set out for the pharmacy dressed in my new scarf, went up to the counter, and handed over my prescriptions. I had brought eight hundred dollars—all I had to my name—but still the cost was three times that. I couldn't believe it was so expensive, and I didn't have insurance because of my Christian Science days.

"I don't have the money to pay for it!" I said in desperation.

"Now, don't worry. If you can't afford it, here's a government number and you can get insurance for your health problems." I'll never forget that man for his kindness.

I went back to the house. Jacqueline was still in the kitchen.

"Did you get the drugs?"

"They're so expensive—I can't afford it."

Without saying a word, she picked up the phone and dialed the pharmacy. "Hi, this is Jacqueline Schnabel. My friend Peter McGough just came in with a prescription. . . .Yes . . . Yes, just put it on my card you have on file." She hung up and turned to me. "Don't worry. You can pay me later."

The next morning, I came downstairs. "How was the medication?" she asked.

"I didn't take it."

"PETER!" she shouted. "You have to take it! Stop playing with your health! You are going to die!"

I went upstairs and took the morning dose. That night I took Sustiva, one of the new drugs in the "triple cocktail." My dreams for the next week were surrealist nightmares, with awful scenarios that made no sense. Someone I knew who was on the drugs told me that would wear off.

I went back to Boston to get chemo for the cancerous sores. Luckily, I didn't have any on my organs.

My friend Paul would accompany me on the four-hour train ride there and back as we looked over his ideas for our friend Philip's apartment, which he was decorating. At the hospital I'd sit in a row of sick people with pale faces and scarves wrapped around their heads to hide the baldness. One very pale woman had my attention. She was so fragile looking. I knew she wasn't old, but the gray tinge of her skin made her look years older. Her husband and their little girl would wait like Paul did with me. After a while I didn't see her anymore and suspected the worst. I was on a Doxal drip that took one to two hours, and during these weeks of chemo my hair fell out in clumps in my comb or whenever I washed it.

When I arrived, the doctor would tell me how long it would take. The one-hour was difficult, but the two-hour one was ghastly. It made me feel like I had liquid fire inside. I couldn't read or even listen to music. I didn't even want to speak. Afterwards Paul and I would go to a food court in the train station. There was an Italian restaurant with a hot buffet that we often went to, but everything smelled horrible. It wasn't the food; it was the taste of the chemo that made me lose my appetite. I'd get a piece of bread to take with me.

I took this trip every two weeks for months. Dr. Groopman was happy with my results and how much better I was getting. I was still at Jacqueline's and was finishing up a silhouette portrait of Allen Ginsberg that Bruno had commissioned. McD was visiting and sleeping on the sofa at Patrick and Walter's apartment uptown. He'd come downtown and help with the painting I was making. We used Jacqueline's daughter Lola's studio at the top of the house. After the painting was finished, McD went back to Ireland.

19

J ane Rosenblum called and said there was an apartment on Forty-Sixth Street and Sixth Avenue above Chivas Clem's that had become available. I said, "I'll take it."

"Don't you want to see it?" Jane asked. I was so desperate I didn't care. But I didn't have any money to lease it, so I went to a friend who had a rich boyfriend who collected art and sold him six mammoth plate photographs for one thousand each. They used to sell for fifteen thousand each. He took advantage of my situation, but now I had money for my apartment.

I called the building manager and gave him the money. It was a slum. A five-floor walkup slum that had crooked, creaking stairs with a beautiful mahogany rail of chipping white paint. It was a mid-century town house between Fifth and Sixth that most likely had once been a grand home.

The apartment was three dirty white rooms with a big neon tube to light up the darkness in the middle room. I took that down immediately. The bathroom and the kitchen were original from the early part of the century, so they were perfect.

I had, over the years, learned from McD how to make the best out of a slum, so I set to work. I reluctantly called Mallory and asked for the rooms of furniture I lent her in Oak Hill. She said no, that she had paid to store it when she moved and wasn't returning anything. I was so shocked by her selfishness that I abruptly ended the conversation. I went to Ricky Clifton and borrowed two rooms of furniture. I had a brass bed and wangled to get the big feather mattress back from Paul, who had gotten used to it. Paul found someone to paint the rooms: my bedroom was blue, the dark middle room was green, and the front room white, to use as a studio.

I changed the wall light fixtures to old brass ones I had. Walter gave me money to buy art supplies. Mostly I would lie down since I had little energy.

But soon, little by little, I was gaining weight.

Somehow, I started to paint again. I made small paintings and then a group of watercolors for a show in Paris. I usually painted in my bed since it was the most comfortable place. I had no means of support other than making and selling artwork. It was 1998, and we hadn't had a show in New York since 1992.

On Forty-Sixth Street I hardly went out and lived in my pajamas and robe. It was too exhausting to go up and down the five flights. I spent most days alone. I could hardly pay the $1,500 monthly rent and many times had to answer the door to an angry rent collector. Through the medication and eating regularly I slowly became stronger. I was thin but not as scary as I had been. Jacqueline commented, "Well, you lost your beautiful head of hair." True, it wasn't the mane I was used to, but by most standards it looked good—if you consider thinning, fried hair a good look.

I was doing better and heard that Dublin had a great AIDS ward in St. James's hospital. I thought I could go back and be treated there since I wouldn't have to pay. I called the hospital to explain my spots and health care. The young woman on the phone had a very thick accent. She asked me to hold on and I heard her call across the room, "Mary, I have a patient with FULL BLOWN AIDS on the phone." I hung up. I thought it was better to stay in New York.

McD came to visit, and everything changed. I made up a little room for him that I had used for storage and set up a single rope bed and emptied the small closet. McD exploded into my life again. He was Mr. Mary Poppins in shambles. He'd do his sewing in the morning, mending his socks and clothes, and washing his clothes in the bathtub. He was in his sun-worshipper mode and would go up to the roof and paint or lie in the nude. Soon, the building super was knocking, saying the hotel guests next door were complaining.

I accompanied him on a trip to New Jersey for him to see a new-age dentist. On the bus was a person from the raw-food meetings who told me that he was off the medications because first his hair had turned white, then it had gotten very thin. His hair was black now, he said, since he had stopped taking the medications and started going to a raw-food healer in Pennsylvania. He didn't look sick at all to me. He kept a lively conversation going with McD as I contemplated his tale.

"What if I washed up on a desert island and didn't have my meds? I'd die," is what I thought. I know that sounds crazy, but at this moment in time, I *was*. I hated taking those meds and I thought that they were so toxic that I would die from toxicity. I took the healer's number, and when we returned to Manhattan I called the raw-food retreat. A woman named Bridget answered, and we had a long conversation. She told me to wean myself off the drugs and take the pills every other day till they ran out. I still had the purple sores of KS all over, including the ones on my face (like the one on the tip of my nose) that I covered with makeup. I followed her advice and slowly started to go off the medications that were, in fact, healing me. I admit I was nuts. All reason had flown out the window.

When I arrived at Bridget's house in Pennsylvania, I was shocked at how suburban it was, and it was right under electrical power lines. Bridget would prepare the raw food for me and for a beautiful young woman who didn't look sick at all. Bridget would eat her meals out. In the morning I'd have to jump on a mini trampoline for thirty minutes. Then we'd both go outside to the back lawn to lie in reclining plastic chairs and be sprayed with water while we baked in the sun naked.

Bridget also had me watch yoga tapes on a large floor-model TV in the carpeted living room. I was supposed to practice but I was much too weak. It was a homemade tape, and I thought the woman doing the yoga positions looked like our hostess but much thinner, and it was. Bridget had a dog that was kept in a separate place, but I noticed his meals looked like the scraps of diner food.

Bridget could tell I was bored, so she suggested a trip to a local Renaissance fair. The fair had wooden towers painted to look like stone castle gates at the entrance. All sorts of tourists in casual dress were walking among the performers. There was a young male contortionist dressed as a jester with jingle bells sewn to his hat. He'd twist his body and bang a tambourine with flying ribbons, engaging the passersby while he twisted like a pretzel. We passed two enormously heavy identical-twin sisters in Renaissance clothes made out of chenille bedspreads who were each devouring a gigantic turkey leg. My hostess looked at me with the biggest smile on her face. "Isn't this great!" she grinned, spreading her arms out as if to take the whole thing in.

"Can we go?" was all I could reply.

"What?!" she exclaimed, and came up to me and placed her hands on my elbows and stood much too close to me, looking up into my eyes. Her thick glasses made her eyes bug out. "Are you all right? Do you not feel well? What's going on?" This kind of attention was worse than my surroundings.

"No, nothing. Just kidding." I was sorry that she liked it so much and that I hated it. She was like a little girl in Wonderland, and I just wanted to leave. "At least I'm in nature," I thought. But the smell of greasy food made me sick.

When Bridget turned to me I'd put on a smile. We went to sit in an outdoor theater while a long-haired, shirtless man in leather jeans swallowed fire and then a sword.

It was time to go as the sun was setting. In the car back to our life under the power lines I could see she was upset. I was guessing it was my lack of enthusiasm for the fair. I broke the ice (mostly out of guilt), saying how nice the weather was. It was a long ride home. I kept thinking, "What am I doing here? I could always go back and take the medication."

I felt guilty that I just dropped Dr. Groopman. I kept thinking the new medications were like the old AZT ones, which they weren't.

So I stayed. But I kept seeing spaghetti dinners in the dog's bowl.

Bridget also had a massage therapist come over. They looked at my skin discolorations the size of thumbprints and wondered if maybe they were alien-operation scars. It always seems to end up with aliens.

The massage was tough. Bridget didn't want her to use oils on me so the toxins could come out of my pores. A weird thing did happen. A sore came up on my leg immediately. It was quite sensitive and turned into a scab shortly. But the massage hurt, and I was screaming, so they stopped—only to begin again.

While all this was going on, my godparents, Cass and Joe, came to pick me up and take me to their house in Philadelphia for a few days. My uncle Joe sat outside. He thought this was for the birds.

The day before my departure I asked Bridget, "Are you only eating raw food?," because I kept seeing diner food in the dog bowl. She admitted she wasn't. That's why she was much thinner in the video. That's why she ate outside the house. I was disappointed and thought about how crazy I was.

But that didn't stop me.

Justin had moved in with an older man who bought a large house straight out of an Edward Hopper painting on a hill near Hudson. David and I would go and see Justin, who we knew had been ill. His protector had taken him on his first European trip, to Paris. Justin brought with him a small old bottle with a cork, and when he went to Versailles, he opened it and filled it with what he called "the air of the beheaded queen." He had it on a shelf with a handwritten note on it, "Air from Versailles." And as usual Justin set up the large new home with antiques, old bric-a-brac, gewgaws, gimcracks, and tattered lace. He created a "Turkish corner" in one room with drapery and a shredded aesthetic-movement chair and an old paper umbrella. He still had the same large pink marble ashtray by his bed. On a dresser he had a vintage papered cigar box filled with broken porcelain doll heads. Everything was beautiful except a hideous kitchen from the 1970s. When he saw us look at the ugly cabinets, he said, "I know it's ugly, but let's not get ugly about it!"

I could tell he was uncomfortable from the many sores burnt off his face. We were used to seeing our friends at different stages of AIDS, so we didn't say anything. He showed us around the house and then outside to admire his pool.

There were Victorian cast-iron planters with palms, and he had planted flowers around a tree. There was a big burn mark on the ground at the end of the swimming pool.

"What happened?" we asked.

"Oh, it had this hideous pool house—it was just a shack, and so ugly. I burnt it down."

"How did you contain the fire?" I questioned.

"The garden hoses!" he snapped. "I sprayed lighter fluid on the sugar shack and threw my cigarette in it. You should have seen the flames!" he exclaimed, laughing. I looked up and saw the singed leaves in the trees that shaded the pool.

I don't remember how long afterward, but John Patrick called me and said he had just come from seeing Justin. Their friend Gigi had called him to say Justin was sicker than ever. John Patrick went to visit and found him lying in bed. Patrick went up to the bed and started crying. "Oh, Justin, I'm so sorry!" Justin put his finger to his lips for silence and pointed to a big Regency cabinet. In it was a TV set showing *The Brady Bunch*. "I just want to see how it ends."

Justin died soon afterward in 1998, and we learned he had a twin brother. We were shocked because he never had spoken to us about him. Justin was estranged from his family. John Patrick told me Justin ran into his mother one day at Grand Central Station. He hadn't seen her in ten years; she had been living in Boca Raton. I had only ever seen a snapshot of her, with sandy blond hair, a tan, a pretty face, and pink lipstick, holding a long cigarette against her pink nails as she smiled for the camera. He approached her as she was walking through, calling out to her, "Mommy, it's Justin!"

She stopped and said, "Oh, Justin—hello, dear. I'm in a great hurry to catch a train. Here . . ." She opened her purse and gave him a small jeweled brooch. "Well, I can't miss my train. Goodbye," she said, waving. That was the last time he saw her.

After suburban Pennsylvania I went back to Manhattan, and McD was still there. He hardly left his bed and said he was depressed. Minette, an old drag queen we knew from downtown, had died, and her apartment was available to us. His depression ended because her place was full of antiques. He'd take off on my old bicycle and ride every day from Times Square across the bridge to Flatbush Avenue, to the ramshackle house where her apartment was. The police had torn the place apart. "It's an old cop trick," McD stated. "They tear the place apart looking for cash or jewelry."

I wouldn't see him till dusk. Returning, he'd sit on my sickbed and tell me about all the queens who'd stopped by to see Minette and how he told them the bad news. They'd usually stay there for a few hours and talk. "Of course, the good stuff was cleaned out of the place," he'd say, "by different friends who thought they deserved the goods." But McD didn't care, because he liked the apartment's "bones" and there was still plenty of Victorian furniture, and an upright piano. Minette was a hoarder and the apartment was packed with old glass and dinner sets. She lived in utter filth, and the kitchen looked like it hadn't been cleaned for decades. The original cast-iron wood stove was collapsing into the floor. In fact, the whole apartment was covered in dirt. It wasn't in "move-in" condition. But McD loved cleaning it. He hired a vegan cleaner to help him. When the fellow entered the apartment and saw its condition, he said, "Too toxic," and left.

Back home David would make me large, elaborate salads to eat for my cure. They were too rough for my stomach, and I couldn't eat them, which would upset him, and he'd reprimand me. I was still following

Dr. Hulda Clark's *The Cure for HIV and AIDS.* Her theory was that parasites caused all disease, and there was a picture in the book of a man who had cured his KS spots. I read later, of course, that these parasites weren't found in humans. She promoted herbs and woodworm tincture, an old way to get rid of parasites. She also had a "zapper" that reminded me of the E-meter Scientology used to test its members. The zapper was thought to pulse low-voltage direct current (DC) through the body at specific frequencies. What Clark's machine supposedly did was kill fluke parasites as one held the two metal tubes with wires attached to a machine that zapped them. I had the herbs, the "zapper," three of her books—*The Cure for HIV and AIDS, The Cure for All Cancers,* and *The Cure for All Diseases* (by 2002 her books had reached over $7 million in sales)—and my raw-food diet. Clark also wanted all commercial cleaning and bath products removed from the home and replaced by ones from health-food stores. We already had done that long ago. McD and I were considered "new age." Among her theories was that hookworms caused depression. I think my brain was made of them. She wrote that cancer was caused by mold in food like apples and bread wrapped in plastic.

I called Dr. Clark's office in Tijuana and spoke to a woman who worked there. She told me that on Dr. Clark's advice, she had had all the teeth that had mercury fillings pulled. I admit I was nuts but not that crazy. I said goodbye. I was out of my mind because I kept on with my raw-food diet. Not only was it a lot of work, but I missed all the delicious cooked foods. Raw-foodists felt fruits, vegetables, and greens were best eaten after being freshly picked, when they are full of many more vitamins, minerals, and enzymes than cooked food. It was still considered raw if one didn't cook it over 120 degrees. McD made delicious little pastries that were not cooked but heated. Sometimes he'd heat them on a radiator. Years later, an In Memoriam website posted that "on the evening of September 3rd, 2009, Dr. Hulda Clark's celebrated life came to an end." She died of multiple myeloma, a blood and bone cancer.

I went to see a Christian Science practitioner who lived at One Fifth

Avenue. I told her I was suffering from AIDS, but she was formal and unfriendly. Everyone at the church on the Upper West Side was friendly (sometimes too friendly, as when an elder at the church showed us the upstairs and kept pinching my behind), but not this woman. I was paying her two hundred dollars (in cash) to read from the Bible and *Science and Health with Key to the Scriptures,* but I didn't return because of her coldness. Later, I bought a book published by the church with testimonials of people who had cured themselves with prayer. I came to the testimonial from a man who cured himself of homosexuality. That's when I threw the book out and stopped attending services.

Just before the end of the century, I ran into Jacqueline at an *Interview* magazine party in the new Dior building on East Fifty-Seventh Street. She saw how sick I looked and knew I was off the meds.

"I can't do it, Peter. I can't watch you kill yourself. I went through it once before. It's too painful to watch. I'm sorry."

I was still demented and determined to show how I'd be healed by diet. In the fall of 1998, Mary Bergtold kept calling me from her home in Arizona, checking up on me and crying each time. She invited me to visit. When I called McD in Dublin, he said there was "the man" out there who would cure me. He was known for healing people naturally. His institute was an hour from Mary. So, I packed my bags and went to the airport. In the airport and on the plane, I could see people avoiding contact with me. But when I arrived in Arizona, Mary greeted me with a big hug. She put me in a lovely cottage in back of her house and brought me fruit each morning and sobbed how upset she was. "I'm taking you to the emergency room now!" she'd cry.

"I'm not going—so stop it!" I'd reply.

I'd sit at her table with her then husband and her two young boys during meals and salivate while they cooked meat on a grill as I sat with a plateful of raw vegetables.

I called "the man" in Arizona who cured people of cancer, and Mary and I drove to see him far out in the desert. When I arrived, he brought me into an examination room. During the exam I kept passing out as he went over my vitals. Mary started to cry. After the exam he looked at me intently and said, "I can't help you. If I'd seen you sooner, then maybe." I went numb and didn't hear anything else he said. Now I truly knew what a fool I'd been.

I was stunned and started lambasting myself for being such an idiot. This was the man who supposedly had helped others when traditional medicine gave up on them, and now he couldn't help me. I raged against McD and wanted to scream and blame him. But no one had held a gun to my head. I chose this insane path. I had read about others who cured themselves and was waiting my turn, which didn't come. I raged against all the raw-foodists.

But I had to calm down and think fast about my next move if there was still time. I was back down to under a hundred pounds, and the purple spots were growing back weekly. When we returned to Mary's, I immediately called my friend Tom Cashin. Tom had done so much AIDS charity work, I felt he'd know what to do.

After I told him my trials he said, "Can you call me back in fifteen minutes?"

"Yes—yes," I stuttered.

When I called back, Tom asked if I could be in New York by tomorrow. I booked a flight.

I went to the address of Dr. Paul Bellman who had the reputation of saving people from an AIDS-related death. By now I was using a cane, since my foot was swollen again and painful. I walked into a reception room full of men in different stages of AIDS, from the healthy to the very thin and frail. This gentle, soft-spoken man sat me down in his office and examined my fragile state.

"I've heard about your diet of raw food," he said kindly. "If you're going to accept me as your doctor, Mr. McGough, you'll have to follow my instructions and let me help you."

"I'll do anything you want," I begged.

"First you'll have to do chemo. We can do it here. What is your insurance?"

"I don't have any. What will it cost?" I asked timidly.

"It will be around sixty thousand dollars."

Tears fell from my eyes. "I don't even have six hundred!" The tears wouldn't stop. I knew this could be the end. I was a swirling mass of emotion.

His sweetness calmed me as he told me not to worry. We went to the front desk, where he asked Gene Fedorka, his very tan assistant, to phone a government agency that covered the health costs for the very sick and poor. Gene handed him the phone. "This is Paul Bellman. I have a patient who needs coverage to be put through immediately." He paused, listening. I could see the agitation on his face. "*No!*" he shouted. "You don't understand! I want this put through *now*! This is an emergency! . . . Yes . . . Yes. Do it now." He handed the phone back to Gene and he turned to me.

"We'll start your chemo treatment tomorrow morning at ten. Don't worry, and just keep eating. You'll need your strength."

I went back to "Little Brazil," laboriously climbing the five flights of stairs, and sank into my feather mattress, thinking about my past and hoping I had a future.

McD called to find out how it had gone at "Rancho Notorious" and what "the man" had said. I told him he'd said he couldn't help me. I then let David know I was back on the meds.

It was difficult to get out of bed, not just because it was a feather mattress, but because I was so weak and any movement was exhausting. I had hired a Bulgarian assistant, Ivaylo, a very sweet master of old painting techniques. I could see in his face that he thought the job might come to an end soon.

I returned to the doctor's office to start chemo. At night I took the drug that gave me surrealist dreams and smoked pot to ease the chemo's burning sensation. I became better each week.

Dr. Bellman kept telling me I had incredible healing powers. A year later he told me that when I'd walked into his office he'd given me only three months to live.

Then I had a call from McD in London, who told me our friend Nina was at a dinner with a fellow from Doctors Without Borders who said there was a woman who could help me with the KS sores by using oils. I didn't want to hear it, and a fight ensued. I told him that I was through with those nuts. Ten minutes later Nina called and spoke to me about this doctor. I listened and then called him. He said that there was a woman in New Jersey who made healing oils. My spots were fading, but they were still apparent all over my face. And I was sick of chemo. I went to Dr. Bellman and told him of the woman. I could handle the AIDS drugs, but the chemo was water torture. Dr. Bellman agreed to give it a try for a week. So I took a bus to New Jersey and waited on a park bench near the bus stop as directed. A large 1980 Cadillac pulled up, blaring disco music. "Are you Peter?" a black woman called out.

"Yes, it's me."

"I'm Sarah. Come on, baby, get in," she said sweetly, opening the car door. Her hairdo touched the car's velvet ceiling, and she was wearing a lab coat. The song on the radio kept repeating "Yawza—yawza—yawzar." Her nails were so long she had to steer the wheel with her palms as her lacquered pins pointed upward.

"Give me three days, honey, and we'll kill all them babies"—the KS sores. "They'll all be dead," she said, touting her healing lotions.

We arrived at a candle store with scented tapers in martini glasses. She introduced me to her daughter, Rose. Sarah's father was an herbalist healer in the Alabama countryside. Since the nearest hospital was hours away, he made salves and ointments for the locals. The mother-and-daughter team kept it going. I was led into a back office that had a massage table. On the wall was a broken clock with a kitten image that read, "Hang in there, baby." I undressed and lay on the table.

Sarah came in and put on two layers of latex gloves and started basting me with a strange but aromatic oil. She gave me a washcloth for modesty. The aroma went through my nose and into my lungs. When she got to my waist she asked me, "Do you have any on your johnson?"

"No!" I answered.

"Okay, honey. Nothing to worry about."

When she came to my feet she noticed some fungus on one. "Hmmm. I got something for that." She opened the door and went into a small hallway kitchen. I watched from the table as she pulled a large clean weed with its roots out of a small refrigerator and put it in a blender, adding some oils. She came in and sprayed it on my toes, then continued to baste me with the previous oil from head to toe. "I'll be back in an hour to turn you over," she said as she exited.

Now I knew how a turkey felt before the oven door closed. I lay there thinking, "If this doesn't work, at least I got a nice massage." Sarah returned and I was turned over. I rested on the table for about five hours and returned the next two days for more five-hour basting. I was instructed to not wash afterward and to sleep in the oils, which turned my sheets and underwear yellow.

After showering on the morning of my second day before I left for the bus, I noticed the sores looked faded. "You're imagining it," I thought. But when I lay back on the table, Sarah exclaimed that they were indeed fading, and her promise of "Give me three days, honey" she repeated. "It's working! I told you so! We're killing them babies." Rose came in to look me over as Sarah pointed to the sores, exclaiming that they were disappearing.

The following Monday I went to Dr. Bellman's and he looked over the sores. "Hmm. It looks like they're fading. Let's give it another two weeks."

I had two creams to take home, one for the evening and one after a morning shower. I kept getting compliments on the scent I was wearing. As the spots continued to fade, that was the end of my chemo.

I didn't know what had become of Bastian, but Ricky had seen him in New York and told him I was sick with AIDS and living near Times Square. I never heard from him in those years of ill health. Since I was getting better, I was working in my small studio in the front of the apartment. The world was getting ready for a new century. We had a show of Bruno's collection of our oil paintings from the eighties at the Galérie Jérôme de Noirmont on avenue Matignon in Paris. Then, just after 2000, we made another show for Jérôme of new oil paintings, which McD called *The Deep Future . . . The Deep Past*. We were making good sales, but not enough to keep both Ireland and New York breaking even.

20

One morning, I received a call from Michael Kors whom I hadn't seen in years. It wasn't good news. He told me Billy Metz was very ill, and if I wanted to say goodbye and see him I had better act fast. I took the train to New Jersey the next day and his father picked me up. Billy was in a dressing room standing in the signature minuscule white briefs he had worn since I met him. He was rail thin, and his once beautiful face was a skull with a thin layer of skin covering it. A loud hairdryer was working the brush on his massive tresses, turning them into a Jackie O helmet as he animatedly made jokes over the noise. I looked at a plate-sized sore covering his back.

He finished his ablutions and laughed as he gave me a big hug. I could feel his boney back. I was still thin, but not nearly as thin as Billy. We sat and talked while his mother made us lunch, like she had done so many years ago before I lost contact with him in my life with McD. Billy had a certain kind of sissy magic like David's but very different. He also was an avid reader. I saw how he had taken over his parents' suburban house on the pond with furniture from his former New York apartment and his Tiffany ashtrays. He had reupholstered the house's fifties furniture in a leopard print and painted the walls bright colors. My painting of his favorite aunt Vi, who worked in Manhattan, was hanging in the living room with some drawings I gave him when we were teenagers. He lit a cigarette with the gold lighter he had stolen from Tom Eyen, the playwright he dated. Billy was crazy for Tom, but Billy was "just one of those things" to Eyen. It was bittersweet to see Billy. He had gotten sober long ago for a couple of years, but then went back to drinking. My guess was that when he heard he had AIDS he went off the wagon.

I felt sorry for his parents whom I knew so well in my youth. Billy was their only child. Before I left, I told him I loved him and gave him a big, long hug.

But after a while Billy surprisingly started to get better and came into my life again. He'd call me wanting to speak or would just drop by if he was in the neighborhood. I'd let him sleep on my sagging divan if he was in New York and didn't want to take a three a.m. train back to his parents'. Billy didn't have many boundaries. He'd call at all hours, and I could hear the tinkling of ice in his drink over the phone. He'd stay every couple of weeks on my sofa, or I'd meet him at some bar in Chelsea. His weight came back, but his face had the look of illness. It must have been very difficult for him to see his formerly handsome face now looking like a death mask. He'd joke and say, "I've painted all the mirrors black."

Poor Billy, he was dancing as fast as he could through life as if he were escaping something. I think we all were. Maybe we were running toward something instead of away from it. Billy didn't wear his heart on his sleeve like me. He told me when we were teenagers, "When I die I want them to play the Eydie Gormé song 'It Was a Good Time.'" And that's what he was looking for.

After a while, I couldn't take the three-in-the-morning calls anymore, with Billy asking to stay over, so I left the phone off the hook when I went to bed. I hadn't seen him for months when the phone rang one morning. It was Michael. "I wanted to let you know Billy died last night."

I was stunned and sat down. "Oh, that poor little thing," was all I could say. I thought of how crushed his parents must be. "You know

Michael, I feel so guilty. I didn't return his calls after all the late-night calls wanting to stay over. I feel just terrible."

"Don't beat yourself up, Peter. We all loved him, and he could drive us all crazy."

After we said our goodbyes I stayed sitting in a chair and sobbed. I cried for the loss of Billy, my other friends, and the crushing thoughts of all the suffering of the ones gone before.

About a year after Billy's death our friend Denis, whom Billy had nicknamed Connie, called me and asked if I wanted to go visit Billy's mother, Flo. I knew Michael had gone to visit her with Billy's ex Kevin. We took the train to the house. Billy had been living on the top floor of his parents' house. After lunch Flo said, "If you want to go upstairs and take anything, please do. I haven't been up there since Billy died."

The room upstairs stood still from the day Billy was taken away in an ambulance. All the plants were dead. Only the stems of what must have been a large flower arrangement stood in a waterless vase with the dried petals on the floor below it. His bed was a mess, and the furniture in the room had been pushed aside to get his body out. The bedroom was filled with his collages, some drawings of mine, and a dollhouse he had been working on for more than a decade. The little rooms were filled with the tiny furniture he collected, and he had wallpapered its dining room with a subway map. I looked over at his stack of Louis Vuitton hard luggage with, on top, a vanity case he loved to carry. On a three-tiered table was his menagerie of porcelain Babar figurines and glass paperweight jewels from Tiffany. The bookshelf was a collection of Babar books and another of his favorites, *The Little Prince,* sitting next to his old copy of *Valley of the Dolls.* I went to his bathroom, which was filled with cosmetics, perfumes, and his hair dryer. Tinkling in the breeze on the tree outside the window were the remnants of painted glass wind chimes we had found in Chinatown. In a corner on the floor was the ceramic Chinese-man cookie jar we had bought one evening on Christopher Street when we were nineteen. I took the cookie jar, a cashmere throw, and the silver lighter he used when he left the gold one in a taxi. Connie and I went downstairs and said goodbye to his parents. I knew Billy's whole family, his mother and father, his aunt and uncle who had lived next door. Now they're all dead. Nothing is left but a memory and part of my story. That was one thing I learned when I was in my sickbed, unable to get up. The world still turned. Life would go on without me. I saw it wasn't going to stop because I was sick and dying. I thought of one of Billy's favorite songs, Peggy Lee's "Is That All There Is?" I now wanted to live more than ever.

21

Eviction notices were sent to all the tenants in the slanting town house. Everyone flew out except me. They even tore off the street door to scare me. But I didn't want to move or look for a new place. I hired a schlump of a lawyer who met me in a Polish diner in the East Village. I held out for a payment of ten thousand dollars that would cover the deposit for a fifth-floor walkup on Canal Street that my friend Chris Brooks owned. I set up camp and slept behind a curtain. McD was in town, and he moved almost the whole kitchen—the refrigerator, shelves, a butcher block on wheels—by the front door to bring it to the street. "Oh, no," I said as I put it back.

Later McD was in Vienna visiting friends we had met at the Champagne Waltz in the eighties. He called to read a letter Bastian had written the Viennese friends—from prison. In the missive he asked them to contact Cowboy Bob to help get him out of jail. David was adamant that we help him. "Forget it! He can rot there!" I railed.

"Peter, we can't let him stay in prison. We have to help him."

I finally relented. I sent Cowboy Bob three grand to go to Florida. My only request for David was that there would be no contact with Bastian.

"I'm not interested in seeing him, Peter."

I called Bastian's mother and spoke to her about getting him out of jail. She replied, "Well, maybe it's good he's there." I was shocked she had said that.

In 2003, when I was living on Canal Street, I received two letters from Bastian. The first was written with a fountain pen on fine stationery, dated in March. The envelope was stamped with bold letters in red: THIS MAIL ORIGINATED FROM AN INMATE AT THE _____ COUNTY JAIL. He started it by thanking me for the estimate on his portrait we painted in Capri and for dealing with the woman he lived with and "the presumably tiresome task of dealing with Cowboy Bob." He continued: "I sense from your brevity of your missives that you do not desire further communication. However, let it be understood that I have often looked back at the unique and pleasant times spent in New York and abroad, and have wondered what became of your career and rapport with David. I engaged in the horse trade, which when coupled with some of the more infamous characters and a penchant for alcohol and exotic older women landed me here." He ended it with: "Please know that my best wishes are conveyed with this letter, from one who is thoroughly and effectively berated and humbled."

I felt sorry for him in a way, but I couldn't be pulled down to hell again.

The same year, in August, I received another letter when he was released. It was hurriedly written in ballpoint. It had no return address. After I read it I understood.

> You cannot know how deeply touched I am by your call, and David's, too.
>
> I suppose you two became my surrogate family when I left school and—as my natural family has quite disowned me— to know you two still care for me even after all these years is so heartwarming. Please beware that all my calls, and the mail, even, is screened, and Carla is paranoid of my leaving.
>
> If you ever speak to Patrick and I could be of any help to him I am willing to leave and take my chances with probation. I will

mow the yard or clean floors or anything for a place to stay and some interesting discourse.

After all your trials and suffering I am so glad you are healthy and have so many friends. If only I could find some type of society where I could be accepted. Certainly, an alternative lifestyle of some sort makes sense, as living in suburbia like this is only to find desolation.

Well, perhaps our paths can cross once again—and if not at least know the silence has been broached and mutual good wishes are expressed.

One day around 2006 the phone rang at the Canal Street studio. I still had a landline and no computer. It was Bastian. He complained about how badly he was treated in prison in Florida, where he still was. Then he said, "I've ruined my life. I'm thirty-three and I have nothing."

I didn't hear from him again until a few years later, when I moved to a 1930s doorman building in the West Village. He called on the new landline and I was so shocked that I dropped the phone and was disconnected. I pressed *69 on the phone and he picked up. "I thought you were mad at me." When he said that, I realized, "Not as much as I used to be." With time I had softened. I thought he had gotten what he deserved. I actually got along with him better on the phone than I ever had. He told me he was living with Carla, an older woman he knew, and her two children, who took responsibility for him while he was on probation.

"You're living with her now?" I asked.

"Yes."

"Are you sleeping with her?"

He paused. "Yes"

"Are you in love with her?"

"Well . . . no. I'm not attracted to her in that way. She wants to get married, and she's very jealous. But it would help me with my parole."

I could see that he had not really changed his ways since when he was in our lives. He asked about David, but I didn't want to get into that conversation.

"Please don't marry her, Bastian. Just don't do that. She has two kids, and you're not even attracted to her. That wouldn't be good."

I heard afterward that he had married her.

Years later, I was looking Bastian up on the Internet, so I could get an image of the portrait we had painted so long ago in Capri. I knew he was in Florida and was working with horses. When I typed in his name, the first thing that came up was a website with many mug shots of him, from a heavy sunburned, dark-haired youth to a worn-out shorn-gray-haired man. In one image out of the dozen mug shots his face was badly beaten. His rap sheet filled a page, from fraud to many other convictions—drunk driving, passing forged bills, credit-card theft. Each conviction led to three years in prison. When I looked at the pictures of him, now quite heavy, I could not see anything of that slim, pomaded youth of our past. By 2013 he was sending me messages over social media.

"Hi, Peter, it's Bastian. How are you? How is David? You look well, by the way—more handsome with age!"

I thought it best not to get involved; I had enough memories. Then, a week later.

"Hi, Peter, it's Bastian. Do you remember racing down 5th Ave in the Model T, late at night?"

Of course I did.

"It was one of the most exhilarating experiences of my life, really, and certainly unique. Who would think that running around in an old car could be so thrilling, so exotic, so very sexy, in the immediacy of the feeling and wholesome of an aesthetic experience. God how I wish I could convey that time, and how it transcended this life into another worldly place."

Then one last message, a year later:

> "I was just thinking of you, and David. Hope you are well. Is that
> an old picture of you, or are you on to some miracle anti-aging
> regime??"

I was on my own hideous decline at that time. I had built our career
up from 2005 to 2008 and was showing with Howard Read again,
since he opened a gallery with John Cheim. Our shows in Paris and in
New York sold very well. Then, with the crash of 2008, I tried to keep
things going with sales and to pay for both Ireland and Manhattan. I
couldn't stand the pressure of all the bills I had to pay. I fired my staff
again and moved to a slummy neighborhood in Bushwick that kept
on changing, just like the East Village and Williamsburg did. I had a
nervous collapse and was forced to see a shrink by my doctor when I
told him what I was up to. I had put myself in dangerous situations,
which usually led to sex with strangers who were on, and willing to
share, their heavy drugs. My dreams were filled with nightmares of
my childhood and being raped—memories I had pushed so far down
I'd forgotten them. My new doctor slid two business cards toward me
over his office desk. "Listen, bitch," he said in his deep Latino accent, as
he stared directly at me. "You're fucking crazy, and I can't just let you
go down that road. I'm not going to let you. I care too much for what
happens to you. You need help. Here are two numbers of shrinks that
can help you. Just pick one. You have to."

I went to see the one who answered the phone first. He was a
good-looking younger man wearing a suit in an office with no windows. At our second meeting, I told him he was the kind of fag I hated.
He asked me why. I tore into him about his husband, his copies of
mid-century-modern furniture, and continued my harsh critique. He
paused, then said, "I sense a lot of rage."

"You're goddamn right there is!" I screamed back.

The first year with the shrink was difficult. I hated him, and I hated talking about myself. I wasn't interested in talking about my feelings. "No one cares anyway," I'd say to myself. I didn't trust him or anyone else. The time after the appointment was even worse than my endless crying on his sofa. On the street everything seemed horrible. The daily rat race loomed large. I couldn't stand the mob running to and fro, gripping coffee cups with their faces in phones. To calm myself I'd stop and stare for long periods in store windows on Fourteenth Street, looking at the ugly, colorful sneakers, trying to retain some of my sanity. I had to promise the shrink each week not to kill myself, since I told him that before I met him, I had stood on the ledge of my twelfth-floor apartment and was going to jump. As I stood on the window casement I heard a voice in my head, "It's easy—go ahead!" Something halted me, and I stepped off the ledge and closed the window.

In 2015 I heard from Barbara, who made the documentary on us, that Bastian had died. She saw that his third wife had posted it online. Barbara wrote to me, sending his wife's reply to her: "Bastian had been ill since December after a nasty fall off a young horse, suffered a brain bleed that turned worse over the winter and passed away in his sleep in the early Spring, March 5th, 2015."

This book was not easy for me to write. I had to relive memories that were more overwhelming than I had thought they would be—not just of my youth, but also of losing friends to AIDS and my own struggle with it, and the implosion of the early life I had built with David. At times I'd stop writing and just sob. Being a naturally terrified person, in my life I had looked for anything that would get rid of that fear, and I found some comfort in humor. In my youth I had always looked for a protector, but unknowingly I became the protector. I had gone from living in a world of fantasy through my childhood drawings to meeting McD, who offered a fantasy of a life that was rich in imagination, but the wrongheaded decisions we made took their toll on us both.

When I was at my sickest, I didn't think of much other than getting well. When I was ill, I thought, "This could be my last day," and when I became healthy again I went back to the drudgery of "just living." In my illness I thought, "I'll just enjoy every day," but in health I went back to my petty concerns and desires.

McD and I were in tune with each other working on the paintings, the photography, and the interiors of our "time machines." I liked McD because he was so unusual. I fell into a life with him, and at the beginning—before Bastian—it was a very happy time, when we were creating a world for ourselves. Of course, we were young and full of energy, especially McD.

David always wanted new experiences. He felt the world was mundane, and he was in search of the sublime. He is strangely brilliant in a way few are, and he is always looking for answers. He never takes things at face value; he questions everything, reads constantly, and is friendly to almost anyone out of curiosity. We often joked about what if we hadn't met. I would most likely have died from drugs and he would be rummaging through the garbage for food. We're like two odd bookends that held a life together.

In the spring of 2015 Vito Schnabel had a show of Rene Ricard's paintings at his Gansevoort Street gallery. Rene, who had died in February 2014, was a very close friend of the Schnabels. Vito had invited me to his mother's house for the dinner after the opening. At the dinner, Stella came over with her friend Alison Gingeras, who told me she was a big fan of our work, and we started a great conversation that went late into the night. She asked me if I'd like to do an exhibition with her at the Dallas Contemporary art museum. I had never heard of her, but said yes. Around the same time, through my friend Aileen Corkery in London, I was offered a show in Ireland at Lismore Castle's exhibition space, an old chapel. They asked me if I knew a curator, and I mentioned Alison. The phone went silent and they asked if I could get her. I thought, "Who is this chick?" Then I found out that she was a well-known curator who had held curatorial positions at the Centre Pompidou in Paris, the Guggenheim in New York, and the Palazzo

Grassi in Venice. I called Alison and asked if she wanted to curate a show of our photographs in Ireland.

"Yeah, sure, I'd love it," she replied.

In May a gay-marriage referendum had been passed in Ireland; and in June, in America, when the Stonewall Inn was landmarked, Governor Cuomo officiated at a same-sex wedding there. Twenty-five years earlier, McD and I had wanted to make a temple to Oscar Wilde. I called Alison and I told her that we'd make a carved statue of Wilde and illustrate the twelve stations to Reading Gaol (taken from newspaper illustrations of the time), where Wilde was imprisoned. We wanted a side altar to the martyrs who had died for gay liberation and another to AIDS; a book in which visitors could write the names of loved ones they'd lost; and a votive stand so they could light candles. Alison loved the idea, and so did the owners of the castle in Ireland. Unfortunately the show was canceled. But Alison didn't want it to die, so she called Dorothy Berwin, a producer who had New York gallery connections, who said she thought it would work for the LGBT Community Center in New York. After many months of meetings, we set it up in September 2017 in the Church of the Village across the street from the Center in a small chapel in a lower floor. We wanted to have it available for marriages and other services.

In October 2018 the show went to Studio Voltaire, a nonprofit contemporary art space in London that once was a Victorian Methodist chapel. They loved the idea, and returned the space to its former glory with a raised wooden floor, chandeliers, and drapery, and even ordered reproduction aesthetic-movement wallpaper. I made the pulpit an overturned wooden soapbox of Fairy soap, and we hung our *Friend of Dorothy* and *Queer* paintings. The first incarnation in Manhattan was beautiful, but the one in London reached the sublime. We finally had a temple/chapel/church for and about the LGBT community. I consider this the greatest achievement of our almost forty years of working because it serves a community. I wanted the visitors to find solace in this place and be able to be married without a sense of being condemned by religious dogma. With both spaces we raised money for homeless LGBT youth. Through this I realized I had been homeless in the first few months of moving to New York in 1978. Since I never had children I considered these kids my own to help. I would never have imagined that this would be possible in my lifetime.

Wilde did not back down in the courts about his own relationships with men and was destroyed. The last years of his life were spent in ill health, ostracized by his circle of friends and the artistic community. That's why I thought he should be the deity of the temple. I wanted it to be called a temple because I thought it best to be a pagan religion. The sculpture we made of him was based on the photographs he had commissioned from Napoleon Sarony for his lecture tour of America. Wilde is an example for all to see as he gazes down from his stand.

A few years back McD's good friend James, who watches over him, took him to a doctor in Ireland. They were caught in a downpour. At the office David removed his wet clothes down to his one-piece long underwear suit with multiple sewn patches and stitches, and hung his damp garbs all over the office to dry. He then took down a painting in the waiting room that he deemed "hideous" and placed it on the floor facing the wall. After seeing David, the doctor asked James to come into his office and explained that David has Asperger syndrome. When I took him to see my doctor in New York, he got the same diagnosis: "He's on the spectrum." That explained a lot for me. It made sense—all his quirky actions and lack of empathy. My diagnosis was anxiety, depression, and post-traumatic stress disorder. And that, too, explained a lot to me. Our conditions crowd our life.

After all the parties, collectors, curators, and critics, the only thing left is the work—that piece of art. All the personalities are forgotten. Art is history. Sure, it's great to be praised, but if one's in it for that, then there's no hope. It comes and goes and maybe comes back. The art world is a much bigger place than it was when I entered. I heard that Louise Bourgeois once said, "Being an artist is not an enviable position."

Our life goes on. McD mostly lives in Ireland still and I in New York. There's a studio in Bushwick, Brooklyn, across from a garbage dump, and I live in a 1905 railroad apartment with sliding etched glass doors in Greenwich Village, around the corner from my first apartment, which Chuck and I shared with a pot dealer in the late seventies. When I was talking to David about our past life in New York, he said, "It all may have fallen apart and come to naught, but what we did, when it was happening, was a great feat. It was beautiful and extraordinary." And it was.

Index

Page numbers in *italics* refer to illustrations.

Illustration Credits

A NOTE ABOUT THE AUTHOR

Peter McGough is an artist who has collaborated with David McDermott since the 1980s. They are known for their work in painting, photography, sculpture, and film. He divides his time between Dublin and New York City.

A NOTE ON THE TYPE

This book was set in Adobe Garamond. Designed for the Adobe Corporation by Robert Slimbach, the fonts are based on types first cut by Claude Garamond (ca. 1480–1561). Garamond was a pupil of Geoffroy Tory and is believed to have followed the Venetian models, although he introduced a number of important differences, and it is to him that we owe the letter we now know as "old style."

Composed by North Market Street Graphics,
Lancaster, Pennsylvania

Printed and bound by Berryville Graphics,
Berryville, Virginia

Designed by Cassandra J. Pappas

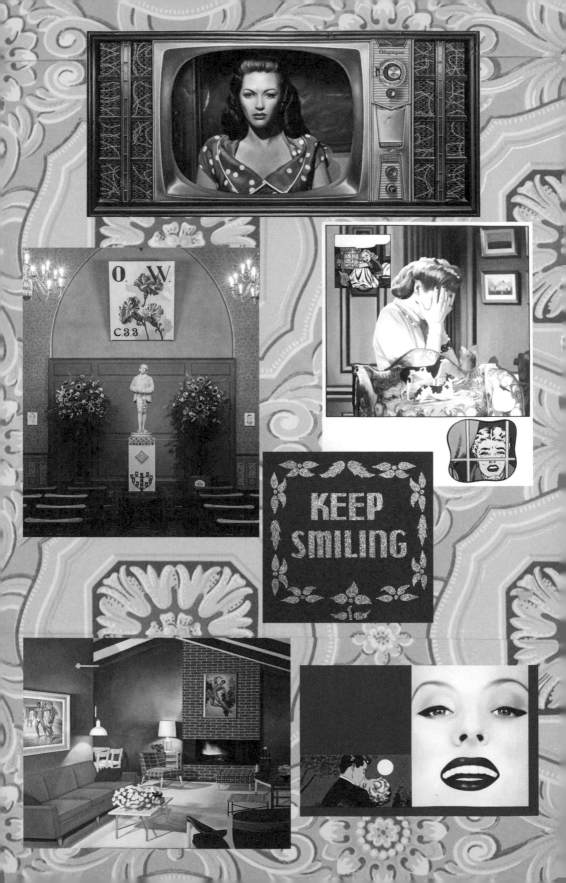